Manual for editors of health science journals

World Health Organization

Regional Office for the Eastern Mediterranean

WHO Library Cataloguing in Publication Data
World Health Organization. Regional Office for the Eastern Mediterranean
Manual for editors of health science journals / WHO Regional Office for the Eastern Mediterranean
p.
Arabic edition published in Cairo (ISBN: 978-92-9021-690-2)
(ISBN: 978-92-9021-691-9) (online)
French edition published in Cairo (ISBN: 978-92-9021-692-6)
(ISBN: 978-92-9021-693-3) (online)
1. Editorial Policies - guidelines 2. Periodicals as Topic 3. Scientific Misconduct 4. Publishing – ethics 5. Writing – ethics 6. Health - periodicals I. Title II Regional Office for the Eastern Mediterranean
(ISBN: 978-92-9021-688-9) (NLM Classification: WZ 345)
(ISBN: 978-92-9021-689-6) (online)

Graphic design by: Hany Mahrous

Printed by: Insight Graphics

Contents

Preface

Health science journals are an important element in health systems. They provide a forum for dissemination of research findings and evidence to improve both patient care and health systems in general. Since the mid 1990s, both the WHO Regional Office for the Eastern Mediterranean and editors of biomedical and other health science journals have sought to raise the quality and profile of journals in the Region. This has coincided with a global recognition of the need for better quality evidence-informed information to improve patient care and health systems. WHO's strategy in the Region towards meeting the needs in relation to journals included, on the one hand, training workshops at country level for authors and editors, and on the other hand, development of the Index Medicus for the Eastern Mediterranean.

Recognizing that this was not enough, in 2001 the Regional Office organized, in collaboration with the *Saudi Medical Journal,* the first regional conference on medical journals. One of the outcomes of that first conference was the establishment of the Eastern Mediterranean Association of Medical Editors (EMAME), a forum for networking among editors of the Region. Working closely, WHO and EMAME identified a number of areas for collaboration, including the need for more sustainable training.

This manual is targeted at editors of health science journals, whether in the field of medicine, nursing and allied health, public health, social health, environmental health or other health-related areas. It is particularly targeted at editors working in countries that are seeking to develop their capacities to promote, conduct and disseminate research and to inform policy and practice.

Manual for editors of health science journals was developed in 2006 by members of the EMAME Education and Training Committee with support from the WHO Regional Office for the Eastern Mediterranean: Ahmed Jamal (*Journal of the Bahrain Medical Society*), Hassan Bella (*Journal of Family and Community Medicine*), Arash Etemadi (*Archives of Iranian Medicine*), Nada Al Ward (*Iraqi Medical Journal*), Mahdi Shamad (*Sudanese Journal of Dermatology*), Fiona Curlet (*Eastern Mediterranean Health Journal*) and Jane Nicholson (WHO Regional Office for the Eastern Mediterranean). The manual was reviewed by EMAME and FAME members and tested in workshops at country level. Subsequent and final drafts were reviewed by Farrokh Habibzadeh (Iranian Journal of Medical Sciences), Maqbool Jafary (*Pakistan Journal of Medical Sciences*), Diaa Rizk (*International Journal of Urogynecology and Pelvic Floor Dysfunction*), Clare Pierard (*International Journal of Tuberculosis and Lung Disease*), Maria L Clark (*The Bulletin of WHO*) and Abdul Ghaffar (WHO Regional Office for the Eastern Mediterranean). The publication was edited by Pippa Smart (PSP Consulting).

Introduction

The past two decades have seen vast changes in the world of health science journals. One aspect of such changes concerns the rapid advances in science, the changes in the field of research in general, and the shift in global focus from "health research" to "research for health". Another aspect concerns the role of journals in reporting research, advancing patient treatment and care, educating health professionals, and helping to bridge the communication gap between researchers and policy-makers. A third aspect concerns the way in which information is delivered and knowledge is shared, an area that has been revolutionized by computer technology and electronic media. One thing that has not changed is the role of editors in steering a journal on its course and selecting content that best meets the needs of the community it serves. How editors accomplish these goals while maintaining high standards and controlling quality is subject to increasing challenges.

The WHO Eastern Mediterranean Region is home to over 300 medical journals. As the result of a drive by the WHO Regional Office for the Eastern Mediterranean that began in the mid 1990s, many of these journals are indexed in regional indexes such as the Index Medicus for the Eastern Mediterranean and the African Index Medicus. An increasing number, although still a minority, are indexed at an international level, such as in the Index Medicus of the US National Library of Medicine, Index Copernicus and the Cumulative Index to Nursing and Allied Health Literature (CINAHL), and an increasing number are being picked up by global search engines such as Google Scholar.

Raising visibility and recognition and reaching a wider audience are issues that concern all journals, but is a particular concern of journals in middle- and low-income countries. Local health science journals are an important publishing outlet for researchers and source of information for the community in which the research was conducted. Therefore visibility at the local level is essential. At the same time editors increasingly feel the need to reach a wider audience, both to share the knowledge contained in the journal and to enhance the global evidence base. Increased global visibility also helps to build the scientific reputation of the journal, in turn enhancing the content it publishes.

The vast majority of journals in the Region are produced in an environment where the resources and infrastructure available for research are low in comparison with other regions, not necessarily because the financial resources are lacking (although that is true in some cases) but rather because a "research culture" is lacking. Paradoxically, as in other regions, academics are expected to conduct research in order to gain promotion. Editors therefore feel under pressure to publish what they may sometimes consider poor quality research while at the same time wishing to improve the overall quality of the journal and widen their audience. These competing demands often mean that editors are unsure of their role and what they can do to address the situation, particularly if they are newly appointed.

The role of the editor encompasses a wide variety of functions which are increased in small local journals with limited resources. The editor is, above all, a leader. An editor needs to have a clear vision of the aim and goals of the journal, and of the constituency the journal serves. The editor treads a line between accountability to the owners of the journal and accountability to its constituency – the interests of which may not always coincide. It is therefore imperative that the editor is independent, both in letter and in spirit, in order to be able to implement the journal's vision. The editor is the ultimate decision-maker with regard to journal content, on issues of concern, and on direction. The editor may also be a manager – of finance, process and people. Many editors consider education to be an important component of their role.

This manual is intended to help editors both in the WHO Eastern Mediterranean Region and elsewhere, whether newly appointed or well established, to clearly define their own individual role, and to set goals and plans for enhancing the quality of their journals. It is intended to provide editors with a practical tool focusing on three main areas: policy and procedures, people and product. The manual can be studied individually as a self-learning experience, or can be used in a training workshop, with all the benefits of shared experience offered by that methodology. While editors form the principal audience targeted by the manual, it is also relevant to and will benefit all those involved in publication of a journal.

The manual draws on the many sources that have become available to editors and the various initiatives that have been developed at a global level in recent years. These are documented throughout the publication and include the following key references, all of which are considered useful further reading.

- FAME editorial guidelines;
- COPE guidelines on good publication practice;
- WAME syllabus for prospective and newly appointed editors;
- ICMJE Uniform requirements for manuscripts submitted to biomedical journals;
- EASE Science editors' handbook.

The manual is divided into three main sections. Section 1, Policy and procedures, sets the scene for editors, discussing the need to establish principles and policies and proposing areas where it is essential to have a clear policy direction. Section 2, People, introduces the main players in the journal publication process and delineates roles and responsibilities for those players. Section 3, Product, describes the essential processes involved in managing a journal and draws attention to quality issues that should be considered. Four annexes comprise additional resources, including SWOT analysis, a list of index services, a manuscript flow chart and editorial checklists.

Finally, the following communities of practice are recommended to editors.

Eastern Mediterranean Association of Medical Editors (EMAME)

Description: EMAME is a non-governmental, non-partisan and non-profit organization whose mission is to support and promote medical journalism in the area covered by the WHO Eastern Mediterranean Region by fostering networking, education, discussion, and exchange of information and knowledge. The Association was established following the first and second regional conferences on medical journals, held in Cairo in 2003 and Riyadh in 2004, respectively. The WHO Regional Office for the Eastern Mediterranean hosts the EMAME web site and listserv.
Membership: Free
URL: http://www.emro.who.int/EMAME/

Forum for African Medical Editors (FAME)

Description: FAME was established by 15 African medical journal editors who set up a professional association and network specifically to review the problems faced by their journals and try to find common solutions. The Steering Committee met for the first time in 2003. The FAME secretariat is at present located in Kenya Medical Research Institute (KEMRI), Nairobi, Kenya. The web site and listserv is supported by the Special Programme for Research and Training in Tropical Diseases, sponsored by the United Nations Children's Fund (UNICEF), the United Nations Development Programme (UNDP), the World Bank and WHO.
Membership: Free
URL: http://apps.who.int/tdr/svc/resources/partnerships-networks/fame-guidelines

World Association of Medical Editors (WAME)

Description: Established in 1995, WAME is a voluntary association of editors from countries throughout the world who seek to foster international cooperation among editors of peer-reviewed medical journals.
Membership: Free
URL: http://www.wame.org/

European Association of Science Editors (EASE)

Description: EASE is an internationally oriented community of individuals from diverse backgrounds, linguistic traditions and professional experience who share an interest in science communication and editing. Based in the UK, it has members from 55 countries around the world, holds a regular conference, and provides a quarterly newsletter.
Membership: Subscription
URL: www.ease.org.uk/

Council of Science Editors (CSE)

Description: Established in 1957 as the Council of Biology Editors, it changed its name to CSE in 2000 to more correctly reflect its membership. The Council provides an annual conference, a bi-monthly newsletter, and an extensive web site and publishes a regularly updated style manual for authors, editors and publishers.
Membership: Subscription
URL: www.councilscienceeditors.org/

Committee on Publication Ethics (COPE)

Description: COPE is a forum for publishers and editors of peer-reviewed journals to discuss issues related to the integrity of work submitted to or published in their journals. It supports and encourages editors to report, catalogue and instigate investigations into ethical problems in the publication process. It provides services to members to allow them to resolve ethical publishing issues.
Membership: Subscription
URL: http://publicationethics.org/

International Society of Managing and Technical Editors (ISMTE)

Description: The International Society of Managing and Technical Editors (ISMTE) launched in 2008 to enhance the professionalism of editorial office staff by providing networking and training infrastructure, establishing best practices and studying and reporting on editorial office practices, ISMTE is an advocate on all issues relating to editorial office operations.
Membership: Subscription
URL: http://www.ismte.org/

1. Policy and procedures

Purpose: To enable editors to establish and maintain clear journal policies in terms of scope, format, management, procedures and ethical issues.

1.1 Why do you need policies?

Objective: The editor will be able to consider what policies are essential to meet the goals and vision of the journal.

1.2 Journal scope and structure

Objective: The editor will be able to develop a vision for his/her journal, and communicate a policy statement covering the aims and scope and the structure and format of the journal.

1.3 Governance

Objective: The editor will be able to advise the editorial board and other governing bodies on the most appropriate division of roles and responsibilities to ensure success of the journal.

1.4 Ethics and publishing

Objective: The editor will be able to establish and implement an ethics policy for the journal.

1.5 Management

Objective: The editor will be able to determine the optimum management systems to ensure sustainable publication of the journal.

1.1 Why do you need policies?

Objective: The editor will be able to consider what policies are essential to meet the goals and vision of the journal.

All journals need to have established principles and policies which guide their operation and ensure consistency in decision-making. This is as important for new journals as it is for established journals. For new journals, establishing journal policies is crucial when deciding why and how to publish. For existing journals it is important to periodically re-revaluate the journal's policies, to ensure that they are still contributing to the journal's goals and vision. Establishing policies helps the journal administration to make the right decisions regarding how the journal will react to challenges and changes, and how it will keep its identity over time.

This section considers some of the most prominent policies, but it is helpful to consider policies for the following items:

- aims and scope;
- process of decision-making for journal policies;
- process of decision-making for individual manuscripts, including peer review;
- editing and peer review of non-article material such as editorials and letters;
- appeals/conflicts;
- authorship and contributorship;
- fraud and plagiarism;
- duplicate submission/redundant publication;
- competing interests (also called conflict of interest);
- advertising;
- copyright and other legal issues;
- distribution models, including free distribution, such as open access online publishing;
- journal funding;
- journal pricing;
- roles of editors and governing bodies;
- scope of activities of the editorial board and structure of the editorial team;
- communication of research to inform policy and practice.

In consideration of the last point, it is particularly important to remember that the purpose of journals is not only to form a communication link between researchers, but also to inform and help influence national and international policies and practice. Indeed, it could be argued that the latter role is the most important role of a journal and supports dialogue between the research community and policy-makers. Developing editorial policies to ensure that the journal performs this role may, for example, involve inviting appropriate people to join the editorial board, or ensuring that the journal provides press releases of important items.

> Can you think of any other items for which you should set policies? Do you have a set of guidelines for how to respond to problems in each of the areas listed above? Who do you think is responsible for establishing policy on the items above?

1.2 Journal scope and structure

Objective: The editor will be able to develop a vision for his/her journal, and communicate a policy statement covering the aims and scope and the structure and format of the journal.

Aims and scope

All journals should have a clear idea of why they are publishing. This could be described as their "mission and mandate". In most journals it is usually presented as their "aims and scope". It is vitally important that every journal clearly articulates their aims and the scope of what they publish. This will provide everyone involved with the journal (readers, authors, editors and owners) with clear guidance of exactly what content the journal publishes, and why they are publishing it.

Although establishing the aims and scope is accepted as a vital part of establishing a new journal, it is also worthwhile from time to time reconsidering the aims and scope of an existing journal, as you may find that revision is required because of changes in your submissions, your editorial board, or your discipline. The published aims and scope are necessarily concise. However, you may wish to develop a more detailed description for use by members of the editorial board and reviewers, in order to help in making decisions about what content to invite and accept.

There is sometimes disagreement about the primary audience of a journal – is it the readers or the authors? Is the prime aim of the journal to provide a certain community of readers with material – or is it to provide a publishing outlet for a certain community of authors? Ultimately the point of a journal is to both publish and be read, but being able to identify the prime audience can assist the editors and publisher to make decisions regarding the scope of the journal and the delivery methodologies. For example, if the journal's aim is to provide information to rural general physicians, then the best publishing model may be a journal comprising continuing medical education (CME), case studies and discussions of new protocols and research, published in print in the local language. On the other hand, if the journal's aim is to make national research more widely known, then the best publishing model may be a journal comprising original research articles, published online in English.

Therefore, to develop the aims and scope, editors and owners need to answer the following questions:

- rationale for the journal – why is the journal publishing?
- target audience – for whom is the journal publishing?
- topic coverage – what is the journal publishing?
- types of articles – how should the journal present its content?

Let us consider each of these questions in turn.

Rationale for the journal

Why is your journal publishing? It is important that you are clear about the need for your journal as this will help you to clarify exactly what the aims of journal should be. For example, the rationale for your journal may be that there is no nursing journal in your region, or perhaps that the prestige of your association would be enhanced by the publication of a journal.

Once you are clear about the rationale for your journal, you can specify the aims (and objectives) of the journal that will meet the rationale. Using the two examples in the previous paragraph, if your rationale is that there is no nursing journal in your region, then your aim should be to provide nurses with access to relevant information. If the rationale is to provide a prestigious journal for your association then your aim may be to provide a publishing outlet for your membership.

Most health science journals would say that their aim was to "improve health care", however this is a very broad aim and you need to be more specific if you are to establish an identity separate from that of other existing journals.

> Spend a few moments considering the rationale for your journal and write this down. From the rationale you have identified, write out what the aims are that meet the rationale. How different are your aims from those of other journals in your country/region? Are there other journals with the same aims as you – and if so, what rationale is there for you to publish your journal?

Target audience

Can you clearly describe your target audience? For this you need to have a clear idea of the public you want to read the journal and the authors you want to write for the journal. They may be the same community, or they may be different. Think about where these communities operate – in which countries, and in what types of areas (rural or urban), and consider their needs and the way in which they want to receive and publish information.

The language of the journal will be decided by identifying your target audience. You may decide that publishing in a local language is required – either for the full article, or for an abstract. It is generally recommended that journals published in a local language should have English titles, authors and abstracts to allow for international visibility. Equally, English-language journals may also find it useful to have the title and abstract in the local language for the same reason.

> Spend a few moments considering your audience. Write down who it is, where it is, and what you think its prime motivation may be for reading your journal, and for writing for it.

Topic coverage

There are many, many journals around the world publishing on what appear to be the same subject disciplines. Therefore, you need to consider what topic coverage provides you with a sense of identity that separates you from other journals, and most satisfies the target audiences that you have identified. What is your subject discipline, and what type of content do you want to publish and provide to your readers?

Spend a few moments considering the topics you want to publish. This may include not only the subject discipline, but also the specialty that gives your journal a particular identity – is it the geographic subspecialty that separates you from your competitors or the focus on a particular subdiscipline?

Types of article

Now that you have your aims, your audiences and your topics clearly identified, you can consider what types of articles you want to include your journal. Most journals would assume that original research articles will be their main content, but do not forget other types of content that your audience may also find equally valuable: for example editorials, reviews, news, short communications, case studies, letters, obituaries, interviews, etc.

It is important to remember that not every issue will necessarily have every type of article. You may wish to set limits on some types of content, such as case studies, for example only allowing one every issue. You may decide to include only some types, such as obituaries, very occasionally, when it is particularly relevant to the readership.

One important consideration to be made concerns translated articles. Increasingly, articles are being published in both local languages and in English. This is considered acceptable so long as the original article is acknowledged and permission is granted by the publisher of the original language article. However, some journals have a policy to only publish original articles, and do not accept translations of published articles. It is important that you set a policy on this issue, so you can make consistent decisions.

Spend a few moments thinking about the type of content that you want to include within your journal – what will your policy be regarding translations? What policies do you need to put into place if you receive a type of article that you had not previously considered?

Establishing a niche for quality submissions

Manuscripts provide the raw material for a journal. It cannot survive without sufficient input. Many local journals in the Region have started enthusiastically with the goal of producing at least four issues a year, but have failed to do so due to lack of material. This indicates a lack of planning and of market research. The potential for a new journal should be studied carefully. If there are too many journals competing for the same material, those which cannot sustain regular publication may have to accept weaker research papers, and will be caught in a cycle of low quality. If there is insufficient research material to support a small local journal, merging with other journals in the country or region may be an option.

To be successful, the journal must find ways to attract the best work from a wide community of authors, since relying on a few "regular" authors will ultimately lead to poor perception of the journal and to isolation. To attract articles, the journal must have a niche or specificity which gives it a unique attraction. Supporting this, the journal must provide a quality service to authors with clear submission guidelines, efficient communication, etc. Specificity can be created in different ways including:

- easier and more effective submission and tracking than other similar journals;
- links with professional societies;
- unique focus on a specific aspect of the topic;
- diversity in the types of manuscripts considered;
- involving the research community through encouraging comments and other feedback from readers and authors;
- innovative format and presentation;
- additional "readable" material such as book reviews, news, letters, etc.;
- speed in publication.

What do you consider to be your own journal's niche? What separates you from other journals publishing in your discipline or region?

Journal structure and format

Once the journal has decided on its aims and scope, this will naturally lead to a discussion of the appropriate format for publishing. Journals can publish in printed form only, in both print and electronic form, or in electronic form only (e-only). Although there are still some communities that are concerned that electronic-only does not constitute a reputable journal, this is changing and it is becoming more acceptable for new journals to publish in electronic form only. In fact many indexes have recently changed their policies and are happy to index e-only journals (so long as they adhere to the other acceptance criteria).

The journal structure is the organization of articles and other content so that readers can easily find what they want to read within the journal. In a print environment the structure can be extremely simple: table of contents then articles. Alternatively, the journal may decide to include "highlights" of each issue at the start of the issue, perhaps selected quotations from articles to attract readers. Perhaps articles will be grouped thematically – for example regional anaesthesia, intensive care, and general anaesthesia.

For a print journal, what structure do you want to put into place? What journals have you seen that have structures that you like? What will work in your environment, and how will your users want to navigate the printed content? Write down a sequential list of the type of content and information that you would like to present in print.

Within the online environment, the structure may be more complex, as users are presented with several issues, and with the possibility of accessing the original data behind the research articles. There is also the opportunity to include additional navigational tools (for example constant sidebar links to other sections of the journal).

When a journal is published in both print and online formats, the situation becomes more complicated. It is not only possible, but becoming increasingly common, for the online journal to differ from its print version. At the most basic level some illustrations may be published in colour online, but only black-and-white in print. However many journals are now including some content in only the print, or only the electronic version, and therefore – in effect – publishing two different journals with a core of common content. Recognizing the separation of online and print editions of the same journal, you are now required to obtain separate ISSNs for each – commonly called an e-ISSN and a p-ISSN.

There are also opportunities to be more creative in the online environment and to present the journal content in more innovative ways. Some examples of how different journals are structuring their online content differently are presented below:

- Uploading pre-press articles, i.e. those that have been accepted for publication and are awaiting selection for the next issue, e.g. see *The Lancet's* Online First http://www.thelancet.com/journals/lancet/onlinefirst;
- Publishing articles online as soon as they are ready, rather than collecting in an issue, e.g. see *PLoS One*. http://www.plosone.org/article/browse.action?field=date;
- Gathering collections of articles in one subject area, e.g. see *The Lancet's* collections page http://www.thelancet.com/collections/neurology?collexcode=115;
- Providing content in other media, such as podcasts, videos and audiotapes of interesting protocols, interviews or discussions, e.g. see the *BMJ* web site. http://www.bmj.com/;
- Encouraging involvement of readers through discussion forums, e.g. see *PloS Medicine*. http://www.plosmedicine.org/article/comments/info%3Adoi%2F10.1371%2Fjournal.pmed.1000072;
- Providing additional content, such as data sets to help researchers evaluate the findings behind the article, and other online supplementary material;
- Interactive CME articles to allow users to check their knowledge against test sheets, e.g. see the *BMJ* e-learning site. http://learning.bmj.com/learning/main.html.

> If you intend to publish your journal online, will it include any unique content – or perhaps the print issue will contain content that you will not put online? What online features have you seen that you would like to implement within your journal? Write down all the elements that you think need to be included within the online journal, and how you would structure these – to help you, visit the websites of journals that you like, and learn from what they do.

Pragmatic decisions, such as the page extent in the printed journal, and the page size, as well as how to publish your journal online, will be discussed in section 3.

Vision

Collectively these components (aims and scope, niche, structure and format) will comprise the overall vision for the journal – precisely why the journal is publishing; what it is publishing; and how it will present itself to the world. Ultimately the vision encapsulates what the journal hopes to achieve.

Resources and further reading

FAME. *FAME guidelines for reviewers*. Kenya, Forum for African Medical Editors (FAME), 2005. Visited 29 June 2009. http://apps.who.int/tdr/svc/resources/partnerships-networks/fame-guidelines

Langdon-Neuner, E. Developing an editorial policy, Part 2: Bringing policies into the instructions to authors or public domain. In: Maisonneuve J et al. (eds). *Science editors' handbook*. UK, European Association of Science Editors (EASE), 2007. Section 1-1.2.

Utiger RD. *Syllabus for prospective and newly appointed editors*. USA, The World Association of Medical Editors (WAME), 2001. Visited 29 June 2009. http://www.wame.org/syllabus.htm

1.3 Governance

Objective: The editor will be able to advise the editorial board and other governing bodies on the most appropriate division of roles and responsibilities to ensure success of the journal.

Introduction

Who is responsible for the overall success of a journal? This may vary according to the different structure and ownership of different journals, but it can be considered that there are up to three partners in journal publishing:

- the editorial board
- the journal owner
- the partnering publisher.

Clarifying the roles and responsibilities of all partners is vital to avoid conflict and help ensure the success of a journal.

Editorial board

The editorial board provides the executive leadership for a journal. The editorial board focuses on the short-term and long-term goals of the journal to ensure it follows the aims and scope statement as closely as possible. Editorial boards assume different roles and responsibilities in different journals, ranging from those of an advisory board that meets only occasionally, to those of a functional decision-making body that works closely with the editor and assists with the daily activities of the journal. This group may have another name such as "board of editors", "editorial committee", "advisory editors", etc. The size of the group depends on the size and the scope of the journal. Possible roles and responsibilities are discussed in Section 2.

Journal owners

The owner of the journal may be a professional association, a commercial company, or perhaps a university or government department. The owner may be responsible for the overall financial success of the journal, and may also feel that it has a vested interest to ensure that the journal serves its membership and policies. It is very important that the relationship between the editors and the owners is transparent, and that each knows exactly what is expected of the other.

With regard to editorial policy, the editor must be free and independent to make decisions regarding the editorial content of the journal. Many journals publish a disclaimer in this regard, usually close to the aims and scope. More detailed description on editorial independence and freedom can be found in the World Association of Medical Editors (WAME) statement on *The relationship between journal editors-in-chief and owners* (http://www.wame.org/wamestmt.htm#independence) and the International Committee of Medical Journal Editors (ICMJE) Uniform Requirements (http://www.icmje.org/#editor). Frequently the editor is employed by the owner, and therefore will (or should) have a contract that clearly states what the owner expects of the editor – for example the frequency of publication, etc.

> Do you feel that you have full editorial independence? Do you have a clear idea of what is expected of you by the journal's owners, and do you feel that there are any conflicts between what they and you expect? Do you have a contract as the editor of your journal, and do you feel that you should have one?

Publisher

The owner of the journal is often the publisher, but it is increasingly common for the publishing to be contracted out to a commercial publisher. In many cases the publisher works in partnership with the journal owner. The publisher may have different priorities to that of the owner or the editor, and as with the journal owner, it is important that the editor establishes what expectations the publisher has of its role. This will involve issues such as delivery schedules, and decision-making levels (e.g. over design). The publisher may also expect involvement in some of the publishing aspects of the journal, for example promoting the journal at conferences, etc.

Do you feel that the priorities of the owner, the publisher (if they are different) and the editor are the same? What are the differences, and do they lead to conflict? If there is a conflict, what can you do about this?

Summary

In summary, it is necessary to define the organization of the journal in detail so that the roles and responsibilities of the editor and governing bodies are explicit. The editor can advise the owner and editorial board on the outlines of their interaction and to what extent the editorial board is involved in editorial decisions. These issues must be included in the editor's contract. The contract must also clearly indicate the editor's independence in all editorial decisions.

For more detail on the roles and responsibilities of the individuals involved in the publishing process, see Section 2.

Resources and further reading

ICMJE. The role of the editor. In: *Uniform requirements for manuscripts submitted to biomedical journals: writing and editing for biomedical publication*. Updated October 2008. International Committee of Medical Journal Editors (ICMJE). Visited 29 June 2009. http://www.icmje.org/#editor

Marcovitch H, Williamson A. Editorial boards. In: Maisonneuve J et al. (eds). *Science editors' handbook*. UK, European Association of Science Editors (EASE), 2007. Section 1-1.3.

Marusic A, Marusic M. Organizing the editorial office and educating contributors. In: Maisonneuve J et al. (eds). *Science editors' handbook*. UK, European Association of Science Editors (EASE), 2007. Section 4-3.3.

Utiger RD. *Syllabus for prospective and newly appointed editors*. USA, World Association of Medical Editors (WAME), 2001. Visited 29 June 2009. http://www.wame.org/syllabus.htm

WAME. WAME *statement on the relationship between journal editors-in-chief and owners*. [Undated] USA, World Association of Medical Editors (WAME). Visited 29 June 2009. http://www.wame.org/wamestmt.htm

1.4 Ethics and publishing

Objective: The editor will be able to establish and implement an ethics policy for the journal.

Introduction

Unethical conduct among the biomedical research community and within biomedical research publication unfortunately exists everywhere and takes many forms. When it does occur, it casts a shadow that can have far-reaching consequences – for example if the wrong information is used to formulate or substantiate changes in policy. It is important therefore that the biomedical profession and the public are assured that research has been conducted within a scientifically accepted, ethical framework, and that what is published is genuine, original research.

Furthermore, authors and readers need to be confident that a manuscript was dealt with in an appropriate manner while being processed. On all sides, a degree of trust is necessary: that named authors are indeed the article authors; that all conflicts of interest are declared, etc. Each time standards of ethical conduct are breached or compromised that trust is undermined. All journals must have policies in place to ensure as far as possible that ethical standards are maintained, and that where they have been breached, procedures are in place to deal with the situation.

Ethics and authors

Conduct of the study

It is important to ascertain that authors have adhered to ethical standards for biomedical research in relation to humans and animals (for example the validity of the research, informed consent, principles of respect for autonomy, non-malfeasance, justice, etc.). Although the journal can only judge the ethics of research after it has been completed, all papers should be assessed to ensure that the research has followed relevant good practice guidelines. Where relevant, the journal should require statements indicating that ethical approval for a study was obtained from a relevant institutional body and that informed consent (whether verbal or written) was given. The journal can ask to see the informed consent form and approval of the relevant institutional review board. In some countries ethical review boards do not always exist, but where they do exist, their approval should have been sought if appropriate. Where they do not exist, editors have a role to play in advocating for their establishment and in encouraging institutions to create them. For example, articles may be turned away if the authors have not followed internationally recommended guidelines for research.

Authors should be encouraged to follow the relevant reporting guidelines for their specialty, and the journal should promote good practice by directing authors to the relevant web sites so that they can ensure the validity of their research. The Equator network provides a gateway to different guidelines, and provides resources for editors as well as authors in their mission to improve and endorse reporting guidelines. See http://www.equator-network.org.

Do you have a policy on publishing good research? Do you communicate this to your authors in your author guidelines? What would you do if you received a paper with interesting and novel results, but which you felt had been produced as a result of unethical research methodology?

Authorship

There are often disagreements regarding who should be included within a list of authors. According to the *Uniform requirements for manuscripts submitted to biomedical journals: writing and editing for biomedical publication*, an author is someone who contributed substantively to the paper based on contribution to *all* of the following aspects of the study: concept and design, acquisition of data or analysis and interpretation of data, drafting or revising the article critically and final approval of the version to be published.

Some journals require all authors to describe their contributions to the work to ensure that they should all be included. A common practice in this Region and elsewhere is that of "gift" authorship – heads of department or supervisors are often included as authors even though they do not fulfil the criteria above. Supervising the research group, on its own, is not justification for authorship although supervisors and other contributors should be acknowledged. It can perhaps be difficult for authors to avoid gift authorship, but if the journal requires a written statement of the contribution of all authors, this may help to discourage this practice.

Some researchers use "ghost" authors to help them prepare an article for publication. These may be what are called "authors' editors" who undertake to rewrite the draft paper to improve the English and ensure that it is suitable for submission to international journals. Other "ghost" authors may be employed by the pharmaceutical companies who have funded the original research, and these medical writers take the raw data findings of the researchers and develop articles from them. So long as there is transparency over the article creation process (both to the editors and the readers), neither of these groups of "ghost" authors needs to be discouraged. The first group provides a valuable service to authors who are not completely fluent in the language of publication, and may help to report the researcher's findings in a more accurate and comprehensive manner. The latter group may provide a valuable service to busy researchers, by reporting their findings faster, and perhaps more comprehensively than the authors would have been able to do themselves. In both cases, however, there are two important points. First, the named authors take full responsibility for the content of the published article, and must approve it before publication, and second, it is vitally important that these "ghost" authors are acknowledged clearly, so that readers are aware of any potential bias. "Ghost" authors should not be named within the list of authors, but must be acknowledged clearly within the article.

Do you contact all named authors to ensure that they comply with the definition of an author? Do you have a policy to deal with problems after publication when either an author has been included incorrectly, or an author has been omitted from the paper? Do you have a policy about "ghost" authorship?

Sources of funding

An author may have been funded by a company/body and this fact may influence the results of the research. While this does not preclude publication of a paper, it should be declared and made clear that this funding has neither influenced the results nor the independence of the author to publish the results or own the data.

Competing interests (also called conflict of interest)

An author may have other interests that could result in bias or improper decisions regarding the research. Again, this should not preclude publication, but it must be disclosed so that editors, reviewers and readers can draw their own conclusions. Many journals require the authors to declare any competing interests as part of the submission process.

Fraud

Fraud is the presentation of faked/invented data, or interference with methods, or selective reporting of data. This is hard to detect at the submission stage but editors and reviewers should be alert to the possibility of fraud. This is serious misconduct: it is a breach of trust and undermines the spirit of scientific research and can mislead readers.

Plagiarism

Plagiarism is the use of work/data/ideas of others (whether published or unpublished) without attribution and implying that the work/data/ideas were originated by someone else (usually the author). This includes self-plagiarism which is when an author re-publishes their own work (or extensive sections of it) without acknowledging that it has already been published.

With the internet, plagiarism has become easier to commit (as it is easy to cut-and-paste content from online publications), but it has also become easier to detect. There are increasing numbers of specialist programs (some free) to detect this form of misconduct, although most of them are designed to work within universities, rather than comparing against other content available online. Some authors, especially those writing in a language that is not their mother tongue, may see no harm in copying text from other people's work as long as it is acknowledged in the citations. However, plagiarism can also hide/indicate a lack of understanding of the science at issue on the part of the authors. It is difficult to say how much can be copied verbatim without constituting plagiarism but authors should be encouraged to express themselves in their own words, not only to avoid infringing the rights of others, but also to develop their own skills in comprehension and writing. If they must quote verbatim, it should be represented as such (for example in inverted commas, and attributed) and limited to an occasional sentence. Editors have an important role to play in raising awareness of plagiarism and in advocating against it.

Duplicate submission

This is when an author submits an article simultaneously to more than one journal. This practice should be discouraged because it results in duplication of reviewing, editing and administrative work and conflict between journals for the right to publish. More important, a study published in more than one journal results in a variety of problems (e.g. biased outcomes for systematic reviews and meta-analyses, citation errors, variation due to editing, etc.), and means that neither journal can claim to be publishing the original article. All journals should make it clear that they will only accept submissions that are not under consideration (or have been published) elsewhere. If an article is rejected then of course the author can submit it to another journal. Sometimes authors feel compelled to submit their article to a second journal if they feel that the editorial office is taking too long to review or publish their article. Therefore, there is a duty on editorial offices to work efficiently to prevent authors feeling this way, as well as to educate them as to why duplicate submission is unacceptable.

Duplicate publication may be permissible in certain situations: for example if the paper is a translation, or if it is of interest to very different audiences who may not be aware of the first publication. In both cases, the authors must inform the journal when they submit the paper, and the journal must acknowledge the original publication so that readers are also kept informed. The authors must also ensure that if they granted exclusive licence to publish, or assigned copyright to the first publisher, they have the permission of the first publisher to reproduce the article.

> Do you provide the authors with clear guidelines about your policies on plagiarism, duplicate submission, etc.? Do you require authors to confirm the validity of their papers when they submit, by confirming that the article is original and not under consideration elsewhere?

Redundant submission

This is the submission of a manuscript that substantially duplicates another paper that has already been published by the same author or group of authors. This typically happens when a research project is written up several times for different publications. Publishing such papers gives undue prominence to the underlying research, and possibly also wastes the time of readers, reviewers, etc. Finally, it undermines the originality of content which the journal publishes, and therefore its quality. To avoid this, the journal should require that the authors declare all of their publications that are similar (or based on the same research) to the submitted paper so that the editor can assess how much overlap there is. It is very tempting for researchers to publish as many papers as they can from their data (also called "salami" publishing) so they can add to their list of publications. Editors should actively discourage and look out for redundant submission.

Competing manuscripts

These are papers based on the same study or data but submitted separately by two or more researchers who have worked on the same study. This leads to loss of originality and there may be issues of copyright if the same content is published in multiple journals. If the analyses are the same then it is up to the authors to sort out between themselves what they intend to publish and where. If the analyses are different, then both papers could possibly be published.

Copyright infringements

Authors may include items within their article that have already been published, and for which they require permission (e.g. figures). To avoid problems, you should require authors to confirm that they have received permission to include any already-published content. You should also note that if an author has published an article and signed over copyright to the publisher, then the author may not re-publish items from that article elsewhere without permission from the original publisher. Many authors are unaware of this, so it is important to ask them if any of their content has been published elsewhere.

It is good practice for the journal to provide its authors with a "permission request" form for the authors to use when requesting permission to include already published items within their article. By doing this, the journal can ensure that it has the rights it needs to publish the items in both the print and the online journal.

> Do you have policies in place to deal with ethics problems relating to authors? Have you experienced any problems, and how did you resolve them? What could you do to anticipate and put processes into place to avoid these problems in the future?

Ethics and editors/reviewers/journal staff

Competing interests (also called conflict of interest)

These exist when editors, reviewers or journal staff have other interests or ties that could inappropriately affect their judgement of a paper (e.g. personal relationship, academic competition, financial interests). All such individuals must be requested to declare any such conflicts if they arise, and the journal should take appropriate action. For example a paper may be submitted by a member of the editor's family, in which case the decision regarding whether to publish should be delegated to another member of the editorial board. The journal must have a policy in place for dealing with such conflicts. If any cases are uncovered where conflicts of interest have jeopardized ethical standards and fair treatment of a paper, then the journal should have a policy on how to deal with this.

Some journals do not accept submissions from members of their own editorial board, or from the journal editor. Other journals encourage all members of the editorial board to submit their best material to the journal. So long as a journal does not exclusively publish articles written by members of its own editorial board, it is acceptable to publish such material. However, to avoid criticism of bias the journal should have a clear policy regarding such submissions, so that the readers can be assured that the decision to publish was based on merit, rather than the relationship with the authors.

Confidentiality

Manuscripts, or parts thereof, or comments of reviewers, must be protected from any personal use by editors, reviewers or journal staff. For example, there have been cases where a reviewer has taken material from papers they are evaluating and incorporated it into their own articles. The journal should have a strict policy of confidentiality in this regard and should ensure that reviewers are all well informed of their ethical responsibilities towards authors. The journal should also have a policy on how to deal with infringement.

> Do you stress the need for confidentiality with your reviewers? Do you have a policy that all members of the editorial board are required to agree to when they join the journal? Are there any other ethical issues relating to editors, journal staff and reviewers that you can think of?

Ethics and owners/support organizations

In the interests of scientific objectivity, integrity and equity, owners/support organizations need to respect the independence of the editor and not influence the content of the journal. The editor must request assurance of this at the beginning of his/her tenure.

Ethics and advertisements

Many journals accept advertisements and may need them to bring in essential revenue. However, such advertising must not be allowed to influence editorial decisions. In biomedical journals, advertising often comes from pharmaceutical companies for their products. A journal must have a clear written policy on advertising, and the editor should ensure that all existing local standards for advertisements that apply to their country are enforced.

Issues that should be considered when creating an advertising policy include the following:

- No advertisements of products proved to be harmful should be carried.

- Journals should not contain excessive advertising especially from only one or two advertisers, as readers may perceive that these advertisers have influenced the editor and biased the content.
- It is not usual for advertisements to appear between articles (they are usually placed either at the start or the end of the journal). The reason for this is that it may appear that the article endorses a product if the advertisement is near a related paper.
- Editors should be alert to misleading or exaggerated claims in advertisements and should reserve the right to edit advertisements – or to refuse to include them.
- The final decision to carry specific advertisements should be the editor's alone.

Dealing with misconduct

So that misconduct can be dealt with quickly and correctly, the journal should have policies and strategies to deal with possible misconduct in relation to all the individuals or bodies mentioned. However, situations may arise which are not covered by prepared policies. If this happens, a wealth of information on how to deal with specific problems is available from the Committee on Publication Ethics (COPE) which also provides useful flowcharts on how to deal with commonplace misconduct issues, such as plagiarism, incorrect authors, etc.

The usual steps to deal with misconduct include:

- request for confirmation of data;
- request for re-writing;
- rejection of a paper;
- referral to the institute the author is affiliated with;
- retracting a paper;
- naming and shaming.

How these can be used in specific cases can be seen from the COPE flowcharts. See http://www.publicationethics.org/

Take a look at the COPE website. Do you agree with the flowcharts that they present – and if not, what other procedures would you use to address issues of misconduct?

Resources and further reading

CSE. *CSE's white paper on promoting integrity in scientific journal publications.* USA, Council of Science Editors (CSE), 2006. Visited 29 June 2009. http://www.councilscienceeditors.org/editorial_policies/white_paper.cfm

COPE. *Best practice guidelines for journal editors.* UK, Committee on Publication Ethics (COPE), 2002. Visited 29 June 2009. http://publicationethics.org/code-conduct

Ethical issues, In: Maisonneuve J et al. (eds). *Science editors' handbook.* UK, European Association of Science Editors (EASE), 2007. Section 1-4.

ICMJE. *Uniform requirements for manuscripts submitted to biomedical journals: writing and editing for biomedical publication.* Updated October 2008. International Committee of Medical Journal Editors (ICMJE). Visited 29 June 2009. http://www.icmje.org

WAME. *Publication ethics policies for medical journals.* [Undated] The World Association of Medical Editors (WAME), USA. Visited 29 June 2009. http://www.wame.org/resources/publication-ethics-policies-for-medical-journals

1.5 Management

Objective: The editor will be able to determine the optimum management systems to ensure sustainable publication of the journal.

To ensure a successful and sustainable journal you need to make sure that you have good quality articles to publish, that you publish it effectively, and that you disseminate it to the maximum number of readers. This requires management of finances and people, and implementation of sound business systems to attract content and promote visibility of the journal to its community. This section will consider the systems that need to be put in place.

Finance and business planning

For the sustainability of the journal, financial issues are important. The editor must have an idea of the resources s/he can rely on, where the revenues are expected to come from (print and online subscriptions, advertising, support from organizations/associations/institutions, etc.), and how sustainable they are. In addition, the editor (or another appropriate person) must monitor expenditure to ensure that the journal does not spend more than it can afford.

Projecting the finances for a new journal can be very difficult, but it is crucial to do this to determine whether a new venture can succeed. With an existing journal it is equally important to evaluate the finances to determine what improvements or new developments can be afforded – for example publishing more regularly, or employing an additional member of staff.

> Do you have a clear understanding of the income and expenditure for your journal? How would you fund new developments?

Many journals are started on the initiative of one or two enthusiastic scholars. This is not usually enough to guarantee the continued publication of the journal. The editor must try to build an administrative body including enough editors and editorial staff. Money and training are both necessary for this purpose, and it is likely that a journal will fade in the long run, or indeed the short run, if it does not have a plan for editors and staff recruitment and training. This is a key issue to consider in starting up a new journal.

Do you have a plan for maintaining skills and enthusiasm from the members of the journal team? Do you have a succession plan in place (how to replace members of the editorial board and the editor-in-chief when they step down)?

For an existing journal it is recommended that you periodically undertake a SWOT analysis (strengths, weaknesses, opportunities and threats) for the journal. This will help to identify areas where it could improve, either by taking advantage of new opportunities (perhaps a new editor), or by addressing problems (perhaps too few manuscripts submitted). See Annex 1 for more detail on undertaking a SWOT analysis.

Have you ever undertaken an analysis of the strengths and weaknesses of your journal? Who do you think should be involved in such an exercise?

The publishing model

With changing technologies and changing expectations, it is worthwhile reconsidering the publishing model periodically. The online environment also offers great opportunity to develop your journal into new markets, and strengthen its publishing operation. Some of the opportunities offered by online publishing are discussed below.

Open access or subscription-based online access

Subscription-based access requires a secure site that only allows access to authorized users (subscribers, plus a list of other accredited users, e.g. the editorial board). It may also offer a pay-per-view option to purchase access to individual online articles using credit cards. This is very common in commercially published journals in developed countries. The disadvantages of this model are twofold. In the first place obtaining and maintaining the secure technology required may be expensive. Second, only paying subscribers (and other authorized users) can access the journal, which restricts visibility.

In open access publishing the articles are published with no barrier to access. True "open access" also allows users to re-use the content (including modifying and re-publishing) without seeking permission, so long as they fully credit the author. There is a great body of argument for online research content to be made open access as it greatly increases the visibility of research across the world. One disadvantage for a journal may be a loss of subscription revenue, however there are conflicting arguments about the actual effect of this, particularly within the low- and middle-income countries. Possible loss of revenue can be offset by charging authors publication fees, or obtaining grant funding. Open access publishing is particularly popular within the biomedical sciences, with many publishers starting to adopt it: for example Hindawi in Egypt, MedKnow in India, PLoS in the USA, and BioMed Central in the UK.

It is possible to effect a compromise between open or restricted access by publishing with either a delayed open access facility, or granting open access to selected articles. With delayed open access, after an agreed delay (for instance 6 months, or one year), the journal makes all of its content available to any reader, with no barrier on access. The benefit of this model is that it protects subscription revenue, but helps visibility by making the content available to all after a specified time.

With selected open access some of the content is available to all with no barrier, while other content is protected and only available to subscribers. An example is the BMJ which makes its research articles freely available to all, but protects its "value-added" content (reviews, etc.) behind subscription-only access. Other publishers make articles freely available if the authors pay a publication fee, for example Springer's "Open Choice" model.

Other publishing models

Publish often online, print infrequently. Making use of the relative cheapness of online publishing compared to the cost of printing and distributing, a model of publishing frequently online, but only printing once or twice a year may be a way to increase your periodicity. In this model the online version could be open access or restricted access.

Publish article-by-article online. Following the above example, some journals have moved another step on, and publish each article online as soon as it is ready. For example, all the journals published by BioMed Central publish in this manner. The benefit to authors is that their work is published very quickly, and also takes advantage of the relative cheapness and ease of publishing online. Some publishers then print a compiled issue (or volume) once or twice a year, whereas others do not produce a print edition unless it is specifically requested (and paid for). In this model the online could be open access or closed access.

Pre-publication articles. Many journals do not publish as often as they wish, which means that authors may have to wait a long time to see their article published after acceptance. To make an author's work public in advance of being selected for an issue, a specific area of the journal web site can be set up to host articles that are waiting for publication. Usually these are articles that have gone through production, and are "held for press" (i.e. awaiting selection and pagination). There is some evidence that this type of service is most valued by authors, and not by readers (except in some fast-moving disciplines), therefore use of a pre-publication site can be disappointing, and be an additional cost to the journal with little reward. In addition, some authors may not want their articles to appear in a pre-publication site, for instance if they have patents pending, or if they are concerned about their article appearing before it has been associated with a volume/issue. Also, you will need to obtain digital objective identifiers (DOI) for the articles in this case, and the work of the editorial office will be increased. The pros and cons need to be weighed carefully.

Online only. Printing and distribution can be a high cost, so it may be worthwhile considering publishing as an online-only journal. A few years ago this was frowned on, but increasingly (particularly in the biomedical area), it is becoming more accepted – for example PLoS Medicine, and all the journals published by BioMed Central. These examples are open access, however there are other examples which publish online only, but are closed access for subscribers only. One point that you should consider is that in some countries and disciplines there are authors and institutional bodies which may still not recognize the online publication as a true publication, making this model unsuitable – but opinions are changing fast.

Have you considered alternative publishing models to help increase the visibility and sustainability of your journal? Which of the above ideas do you think would be appropriate for your journal? What other ideas do you have to take advantage of new publishing models?

Promotion of the journal

It is unrealistic to expect that a journal will naturally become well known – even if it is publishing high quality material. To raise the visibility of a journal outside its own small community takes effort, but it is well worth the investment of time and resources. It does not require large budgets to promote a journal, but it does take some imagination and time.

The prime audience to which a journal must promote itself is to potential new authors, so that it will attract the high quality manuscripts which are vital to increasing journal use and impact. Frequently, both readers and authors form part of the same community, so by promoting to one community, you automatically reach the other.

In planning promotional activities the editor must have a clear idea of the audience s/he is targeting. Defining the target audience can prevent the editor from wasting resources and energy on activities that do not lead to effective journal promotion.

A journal can build a good reputation with its authors by providing good services, such as:

- working with authors and taking an active role in producing good manuscripts: this can be done in the form of effective review reports, training workshops, etc.;
- providing good, clear, concise author guidelines;
- defining and maintaining high publishing standards: this can be done through using trained professional staff, language editors, methodological advisers, and internal reviewers;
- developing an effective online submission and tracking system which helps authors to submit, reviewers to review and editors to oversee the process;
- defining and maintaining high standards of effective editorial process: thorough peer review, speed of decision-making, quality of proofs before publication, etc.;
- increasing visibility to the target readers: online and print versions with timely and effective distribution, presence in libraries, indexing in bibliographic databases.

A journal can promote its content to prospective readers (and authors) through activities such as:

- working with other journals by exchanging journals, editors, reviewers etc.;
- collaborating with other journals to exchange abstracts, supply each other's subscribers with copies of the journal, etc.;
- making good use of the editorial board to act as journal representatives and attract contributions;
- providing the editorial board with a supply of leaflets to hand out at meetings;
- attending conferences and meetings;
- asking members of the editorial board to include their position on the journal as part of their e-mail "signature";
- working with large professional publishers where appropriate;
- ensuring the journal is included within the relevant indexes (see below);
- signing agreements with subscription agents to promote and sell the journal abroad;
- exchanging advertisements with other journals;
- sending out calls for papers for themed issues;
- e-mailing target groups with information about the latest issue;
- providing e-mail table-of-contents alerts.

More detailed description of journal promotion methods can be found in the EASE Science Editors' Handbook – see the reference at the end of this section.

Having a policy for journal dissemination helps the journal reach its audience. As already mentioned, defining this target audience is crucial, since it determines the circulation of the journal.

Examples of such target audiences include:

- professionals and researchers;
- libraries;
- societies and institutions;
- other journals;
- companies;
- hospitals;
- government officials.

Strategies to reach this audience can include:

- subscription;
- complementary copies;
- online full text articles;
- including journal web site link in editors' correspondence;
- providing leaflets, posters, and other promotional material;
- e-mail alerts including table of contents;
- posters at conferences and professional meetings.

What other means of promotion to authors, librarians and readers can you think of? What promotion have you undertaken that you thought was particularly successful – what have you learnt from this?

Indexing

One of the major challenges for journals is getting more visibility through indexing in bibliographic databases. There are generally three categories of such databases:

- general international indexes (such as Web of Knowledge, H.W. Wilson);
- specialized/topic-oriented indexes (such as Medline, Embase, Chemical Abstracts, Toxline);
- local/geographic indexes (such as Index Medicus for Eastern Mediterranean Region [IMEMR], African Index Medicus, African Journals OnLine [AJOL], national indexes.).

All indexes have some minimal requirements for inclusion. Depending on the vision of the indexing service, they may set strict criteria on content (for example Web of Science), or be more inclusive but require other qualifications such as geographical location (like local indexes). The most common criteria include the following.

- Quality of editorial work
  - uniformity, and the presence of journal house style for different parts and types of manuscripts;
  - informative journal title;
  - fully descriptive article titles and abstracts;
  - complete bibliographic information for all cited references;
  - address information for authors;
  - application of the peer review process;
  - adherence to ethical guidelines for conduct of research.
- Production quality
  - timeliness of publication;
  - quality of the layout, printing, graphics and illustrations.
- Content
  - emerging topics;
  - "hot fields" in the literature;
  - validity, importance, originality and contribution to coverage of the field;
  - predominance of original and state-of-the-art review articles rather than reprints and translations.
- Language requirements
  - although many journals are published in other languages, English article titles, abstracts, and keywords are required by many indexes.

- Diversity
  - diversity among authors of both source articles and cited articles;
  - diversity of authors' affiliations.

Journals must have a plan for getting indexed. It may be appropriate for a new journal to seek inclusion in the country index as soon as they start publishing, but not to seek indexing in some of the more specialist indexes until they have become more established, and can prove that they meet the requisite criteria. For example some indexes require a minimum number of issues, or a time period between applications. Most indexing services provide fact sheets indicating details of their inclusion criteria. Some of the more well known indexing services are listed in the Annex 2 including the Index Medicus for the Eastern Mediterranean Region (IMEMR), which indexes peer-reviewed journals from the countries covered by the WHO Eastern Mediterranean Region, and the African Index Medicus which indexes peer-reviewed African journals.

Is your journal included in any national or international indexes?
Do you have a plan for obtaining inclusion?

Editorial office operations

The success of a journal involves not only good science, but also efficient management of the publication process. In particular, managing the flow of submitted or commissioned articles is crucial to success. This includes routine office tasks – managing the flow of manuscripts and other documents, storing and accessing information, and monitoring and evaluating the processes. Systems for these processes must be put in place and managed. If possible, it is advisable to have a full time manager for the editorial office so that the editor can focus on editing tasks. The manager will ideally be familiar with the journal topic and also have some editorship abilities.

While it may not be easy to find support staff with previous experience of working for a science journal, especially in developing countries, many of the functions involved are comparable to those of any office. In an institutional setting, such as a university, there should be no difficulty finding interested support from graduates and faculty. Generally speaking, the following functions are necessary, while there need not be one person for each task:

- administrative support (secretarial/clerical);
- language/copy editor;
- technical editor;
- graphic designer or illustrator;
- publishing technician;
- computer technician.

Running the journal office needs hardware, software and other equipment in order to operate professionally. Even if these are not available at first, the editor can make a list of such requirements to establish priorities and needs in the future. The list must take into account space requirements and equipment, such as tables and chairs, computers, software, internet connections, telephone, fax, etc.

The processes inside a journal's office can be divided into three major categories: routine office work and correspondence, manuscript handling and production. Although parts of each of these activities might be done outside the office, the task of final supervision and quality control should be the responsibility of the office team, which is in turn supervised by the editor and his/her appointed manager. Thus, preparing a detailed manual of operations for the office is a useful tool to ensure that all members of the team know their roles, and will help free the editor to concentrate on the content of the journal.

What resources do you have to operate the editorial office? Are people's roles clearly defined?

Manuscripts can be received in three different ways; on paper, online or by email. Many journals now prefer either of the last two, due to ease and speed and the fact that it facilitates review and production processes. Online submission systems (also sometimes called "peer review software" or "article management software") are becoming more common, but any decision on implementing such systems, apart from feasibility issues, must take into account the costs of establishing and managing them. There are some open source software programmes available, but their use and implementation may need technical assistance. A good example of an open source system is Open Journal Systems (http://pkp.sfu.ca/?q=ojs). There is also a range of commercial systems.

It can help understanding of the processes if a flow diagram of the manuscript handling processes is drawn up. This should include the person(s) responsible for each stage, the stages from submission to final acceptance or rejection, showing the communication steps of the editor, the board, the reviewers, etc., and the correspondence necessary at each point, deadlines for each stage, and the reports to be given to the editor or the manager. A simple example is given in Annex 3.

The process can best be handled with an efficient editorial management software and database, but in the absence of such software, an organized paper-based registration and follow-up system might serve the purpose just as well for a small or mid-sized journal. As the journal grows, the use of a computer-based searchable database and management system becomes more necessary.

To make communication more efficient, it is worthwhile setting up a series of correspondence templates, preferably more than one for each purpose, to ease the task of composing the right letter at the right time. Some of the usual correspondence templates include:

- acknowledgment of receipt (original and revised versions), to authors;
- enquiry about availability to review, to reviewers;
- letter with reviewing instructions, to reviewers;
- request for revision, to authors;
- decision letters (rejection, acceptance, conditional acceptance), to authors;
- request for clarification regarding copyright, ethical/institutional review board approval, authorship etc., to authors;
- feedback, to reviewers.

Timeliness is very important in the editorial office. One person should be responsible for tracking the manuscripts from one stage to another, and the editor should be able to get a clear image of what manuscripts are in progress, and at what stage, whenever necessary (in addition to routine reports). The editor must also relay the necessary information to the authors in a timely fashion. The tracking method should be mentioned in the instructions to authors and they should be given an indication of when to expect feedback from the journal.

At the end of the manuscript handling process, the accepted material enters the production process.

> Do you have systems in place to monitor and evaluate your editorial office processes? Can you identify more efficient processes that would help the office operate more smoothly?

Establishing a peer review system

The quality of a journal depends on the quality of its content, and reviewers play a vital role in advising the editor. You should not over-burden reviewers with manuscripts which have no prospect of being published, and therefore it is advisable to have an internal review process before sending papers out to reviewers. The internal review aims to quickly ascertain if the manuscript fits within the journal's aim and scope, if it has the essential elements of a scientific article, if the author has followed the instructions to authors, and if the article is comprehensible. While poor language skills alone should not prevent further review, the scientific content must be understandable for review purposes. The editor, associate editors or the manager can be responsible for the task of internal review.

The first step in establishing a peer review system is to define the review policy. There are three basic models:

- double-blind review: neither the reviewers nor the authors know each other's identity;
- single-blind review: the reviewers know the identity of the authors, but the authors do not know who the reviewers are;
- open review: both authors and reviewers know each other's identity.

Most journals adopt the first or second, while others are starting to operate an open reviewing system. Whether or not blinding improves review quality and reduces bias has been the subject of much debate (see the *JAMA* article in the Resources and further reading section below), but in the end it seems that some communities of editors, authors and especially reviewers are "uncomfortable" with open review systems. It is up to the journal editor to decide, in the setting of a particular journal, which system would best ensure scientific integrity and cooperation. Once a policy is chosen, it should be made clear in the instructions to authors and reviewers.

Several journals are experimenting with different types of review, such as publishing the reviewers' comments with the manuscript. To see some of the experiments, look at the Association of Learned and Professional Society Publishers (ALPSP) "Hot topics" web page on Editing issues (http://HotTopics.alpsp.org).

Examples of different types of peer review include:

- open review, e.g. all BioMed Central medical journals, *BMJ*;
- open peer review and publication: all articles are published if authors obtain three reviews from the editorial board, which are published next to the amended article, e.g. *Biology Direct*;
- two-stage internal and community peer review: editors ensure the basic scientific and technical quality, then upload article for open review, e.g. *PLoS One*;
- three-stage internal and community peer review: first, a closed traditional review followed by author revision; then the online pre-print is published for user comments, followed by author revision; finally, editorial decision and publication, e.g. *Journal of Interactive Media in Education*;
- peer review consortium: if one journal rejects, then other journals in the consortium will accept the peer review comments to avoid requiring further peer review, e.g. a group of neuroscience journals (http://nprc.incf.org).

While it is quite acceptable for a peer reviewed journal to only peer review original articles (including review articles), some journals also externally review content such as letters, editorials and even advertisements. However, this is probably to be discouraged (unless the editor particularly wants external opinion), as it may overburden the willing reviewers.

Once you have decided which process of peer review to adopt, the journal must set up a searchable database of reviewers. This database could be as simple as an indexed address book, or become part of the editorial and submission database. Many editorial management systems incorporate such information.

What system of peer review do you operate? Have you considered any of the alternative systems? Do you think any of them would help you to obtain good feedback and improve the papers that you publish?

It is useful to establish written criteria for the selection of reviewers, and it is worth keeping in mind that younger researchers, although less well qualified or experienced, often produce the best reviews. The FAME guideline on selecting reviewers is a useful resource for such selection (http://apps.who.int/tdr/svc/resources/partnerships-networks/fame-guidelines).

Manuscripts can be reviewed by editor(s), the editorial board or external reviewers. It is usual to send manuscripts to a minimum of two external reviewers so that balanced feedback can be obtained. Some papers may need to be evaluated by different people in different specialties. Original articles may also need to be reviewed by a biostatistician to assess the methodology and statistical analyses. Online review systems facilitate the communication between editors and reviewers and potentially increase the speed of peer review. Online submission systems usually include a reviewing system to allow the entire process from submission to final decision to take place online, e.g. Open Journal Systems (http://pkp.sfu.ca/?q=ojs).

It is recommended that journals monitor the performance of their reviewers periodically. Some journals apply a rating system to maintain an up-to-date list of those reviewers who are most thorough and reliable. A checklist for reviewer evaluation will help in choosing more effective and helpful reviewers in the future. Results of this checklist can be kept in the reviewers' database as the profile of each reviewer. Examples of items that can be included in reviewers' evaluation are:

- timeliness;
- ease of communication;
- depth of the review;
- clear and instructive comments;
- positive attitude;
- lack of bias;
- willingness to cooperate.

A useful reviewer evaluation form can also be found among the FAME tools (http://apps.who.int/tdr/svc/resources/partnerships-networks/fame-guidelines).

> How many reviewers do you have in your database? Do you have a system to increase your database of reviewers? How do you evaluate their performance?

To avoid overburdening a small group, the editor and the editorial board should always be looking for new reviewers. Experts, though very knowledgeable and experienced, may not have enough time to read and review a manuscript in depth, and it is a good idea to recruit young reviewers, as well as to retain more experienced reviewers to serve as editorial advisers or reviewers of more complicated papers.

Ways of enlarging your database of reviewers include:

- asking colleagues;
- asking the authors to suggest names of reviewers;
- searching suitable databases (e.g. PubMed) to identify people working in the same area;
- asking members of the editorial board to suggest new people;
- asking respected reviewers to suggest and mentor new (young) reviewers;
- using the reference lists in the articles; the e-mail addresses of many of the authors can be found on the internet.

Training of reviewers (if possible) may help not only to increase the quality of the reviewing but also to improve the submitted papers. Editors will usually not have the resources to run training programmes for their reviewers alone, but may be able to undertake such activities jointly in association with other editors or organizations.

To support your reviewers, the journal should have a review form (guidelines for reviewers) to be sent to the reviewer. It is helpful to both the reviewer and the journal to provide such guidance, rather than expecting the reviewer to create an independent response (which may be difficult to compare with another review of the same paper).

Samples of such forms and other guidance can be found on some journal web sites.

- See the journal *Ophthalmology* for an example of such a form, plus a reviewer evaluation system: http://www.ophsource.org/periodicals/ophtha/content/peer_review
- The *Annals of Emergency Medicine*, provides useful examples of good reviews, plus guidelines in their "Instructional Guide for Peer Reviewers of Biomedical Manuscripts": http://www3.us.elsevierhealth.com/extractor/graphics/em-acep/
- A FAME tool is available as another example: http://apps.who.int/tdr/svc/resources/partnerships-networks/fame-guidelines
- *BMJ* also provides useful information on its web site: http://resources.bmj.com/bmj/reviewers/

Reviewers should be asked to keep information in the manuscript confidential. This includes not discussing the content with other colleagues, not making use of the content or citing it before publication and not making or keeping a copy of the unpublished manuscript. Reviewers should also be encouraged to send their reports on time. Timeliness is not always achieved by giving reviewers more time than necessary, and it is often better to ask for a review within a short period of time than to give a long time. The journal office should contact the reviewers near the deadline, reminding them of the approaching time limit. It is not uncommon for a reviewer to fail to respond, in which case an additional reviewer needs to be found as soon as possible.

Reviewers are, in a broad sense, also "customers" of the journal (other customers include authors and readers.) They are essential to the journal in maintaining its scientific integrity and pursuing its goals. In order to expect timely and efficient reviews, a few principles must be observed.

- It is important not to overload good reviewers. Many journals inadvertently "punish" good and timely reviewers by bombarding them with more manuscripts. A maximum of four per year is advised.
- It is polite for the journal to ask the potential reviewer if s/he is willing and has the time to do the review before sending them a manuscript. Besides showing respect for the reviewer's time and opinion, this will reduce the number of unanswered reviews and speed up the manuscript evaluation process.
- Reviewers should be thanked for their work.

Giving feedback to reviewers will help them feel part of a team, and encourage them to take more active roles. Feedback can be in the form of a simple acknowledgment of receipt of review, thanking reviewers if they provide an especially helpful review or review a particularly challenging paper, asking their opinion about the final decision on a manuscript they have already reviewed, and letting them know how their review has affected the decision.

Other ways to involve and encourage good reviewers include asking their opinion about the review process and journal policies, and formally thanking them by mentioning their names (without specifying manuscripts they have reviewed, if the journal has a blind review policy) in (usually) the last issue of a volume. A few journals create material incentives for the reviewers, such as a free (perhaps online) subscription to the journal, or supplying them with a promotional item from the journal, such as a pen. Not all journals have the resources to do this, and not all reviewers find such incentives an important or even positive gesture. However, if a journal does have the resources, it can make the reviewers feel valued if some of the best ones are thanked in some formal manner.

How do you thank reviewers for improving the quality of what you publish? Can you think of ways to thank them that the journal can afford and which would be appreciated by your reviewers?

Resources and further reading

FAME. *FAME guidelines for reviewers*. Kenya, Forum for African Medical Editors (FAME), 2005. Visited 29 June 2009. http://apps.who.int/tdr/svc/resources/partnerships-networks/fame-guidelines

INASP. *Publishing workshop materials*. UK, International Network for the Availability of Scientific Publications, 2005. Visited 29 June 2009. http://www.inasp.info/file/e03e0ce7ca5d2c6dd8fa7ba722624630/publisher-workshops.html

Jefferson T et al. Effects of editorial peer review: a systematic review. *JAMA*, 2002, 287(21): 2784-2786.

Marusic A, Marusic M. Promotion of journals, especially small scholarly journals. In: Maisonneuve J et al. (eds). *Science editors' handbook*. UK, European Association of Science Editors (EASE), 2007. Section 4-3.3.

Marusic A, Marusic M. Organizing the editorial office and educating contributors. In: Maisonneuve J et al. (eds). *Science editors' handbook*. UK, European Association of Science Editors (EASE), 2007. Section 4-3.2.

Utiger RD. *Syllabus for prospective and newly appointed editors*. USA, World Association of Medical Editors (WAME), 2001. Visited 29 June 2009. http://www.wame.org/syllabus.htm

2. People

Purpose: To enable editors to develop and maintain effective interaction with and between the editorial team, authors, reviewers and readers.

2.1 Editorial team

Objective: The editor will be able to define the individual roles of members of the editorial team.

2.2 Authors

Objective: The editor will be able to prepare and publish clear instructions for authors and establish effective mechanisms for communication and interaction with authors

2.3 Reviewers

Objective: The editor will be able to prepare guidelines for reviewers, develop a plan to encourage good and timely reviews, and develop a plan to attract new reviewers.

2.4 Readers

Objective: The editor will be able to develop a plan to enhance the readership of the journal and encourage feedback from readers.

2.5 Publishers, owners or sponsoring society

Objective: The editor will be able to clarify and develop strong working relationships with the publishers, owners or the sponsors of the journal.

2.1 Editorial team

Objective: The editor will be able to define the individual roles of members of the editorial team.

The editorial team comprises several roles. The principal roles are described in this section together with their attendant responsibilities.

Editor-in-chief/editor

The editor is the steward of the journal. S/he provides direction for the journal and is responsible for building a strong management team. S/he must consider and balance the interests of readers, authors, staff, owners, editorial board members, advertisers and the media.

As the editor is ultimately responsible for the content of the journal, s/he must be a well qualified scientist and a competent researcher, and well respected within her/his field. Ideally s/he should already have experience of, and been actively involved in the process of reviewing and editorial duties, and have personal expertise and knowledge of the journal's subject, as well as experience as an author. S/he must have understanding of scientific methodology and critical analysis skills.

The editor is accountable to the owners of the journal, as well as other stakeholders. Support should be provided by the owners to the editor and the team to develop the journal and develop their capacities and skills in editorship. Such support could include attendance at courses and scientific meetings.

When an editor is appointed, a contract should be drawn up detailing the terms and conditions of their position, and the term (length) of appointment, and including an explicit written statement from the journal's owner that defines the editor's rights and autonomy.

Role and responsibilities

The editor can be considered to be the "chief executive officer" (and may sometimes be called the "executive editor") of a journal, as s/he is ultimately responsible for what is published in the journal, and the success and efficiency of the publishing process. Her/his role and responsibilities may extend to include items that are listed under other members of the editorial team.

The editor is expected to:

- set and/or review with members of editorial board the journal's policies, including those regarding authorship, peer review, quality control and ethical issues;
- monitor and maintain agreed policies;
- ensure that the journal's processes are transparent to stakeholders;
- take final responsibility for the editorial content of the journal;
- maintain editorial independence;
- make final decisions on manuscripts;
- manage and organize the editorial office and ensure good working practice;
- attract authors to submit quality manuscripts to the journal;
- try to develop the journal in every way possible;
- plan for the future of the journal;
- represent the journal in national and international forums.

Do you agree with these responsibilities? Are there any other responsibilities that you feel the editor-in-chief should be expected to undertake? Spend a few moments listing what you consider to be the primary roles and responsibilities of the editor.

Associate editors

These are the members of the editorial team who assist the editor in conducting his/her editorial duties or to whom the editor delegates certain tasks. They are usually appointed by the editor or elected by the editorial board, and not usually by the owner. However, for some journals that are owned by an association, the owner may sometimes request that certain members of the association join this team. Associate editors work closely with the editor to help maintain the quality of the journal and provide support when difficult decisions need to be made – for example ethical problems. The number of associate editors depends on the size of the journal. There may be just one, or a team of six or ten, depending on the journal. They are usually senior professionals or scientists who have experience of publishing (either as authors, editors or reviewers), and are usually fully employed in their professional role, and only work on the journal on an occasional basis. Sometimes the group of associate editors is called the "editorial panel".

Role and responsibilities

Commonly, associate editors are specialists in one particular area of the journal, and they take responsibility for that area: for example there may be one associate editor who deals with the continuing medical education (CME) material, or perhaps one who deals with case studies. It is common in some disciplines to have a statistical editor, who takes particular responsibility for checking this type of content in submitted papers. When a journal publishes on a wide range of topics (for example a general medicine journal), there may be a large number of associate editors, who each deal with a particular specialty, for example oncology, neurology, etc.

Associate editors are usually expected to:

- assist the editor in implementing the policies of the journal and in monitoring the efficiency of its systems;
- correspond and work with authors and reviewers;
- review and revise papers for quality and relevance;
- recommend a course of action for submitted manuscripts in their specialist area.

> Do you have associate editors for your journal? If not, what support can you draw on? Spend a few moments listing what you consider to be the primary roles and responsibilities of the associate editors.

Assistant editors

These are usually more junior members of the editorial team who assist the editor in conducting the editorial duties or to whom the editor delegates certain tasks. They are usually appointed by the editor or elected by the editorial board, but may be appointed by the owner. Their work is critical for maintaining the quality of the journal, and they need to be highly proficient in running an editorial office and good at dealing with authors and reviewers. They should have a general understanding of the subject area of the journal, but they do not need to be specialists in the area. Depending on the size of the journal, this position may be filled by a part-time person, or the journal may have one or more full-time assistant editors. In an academic setting, assistant editors are often interested graduate students or junior faculty. In small journals this work is often undertaken by an administrator or secretary. Sometimes this role is undertaken by someone who provides more than administrative support to the editor, and who can also make initial decisions on whether papers are suitable for consideration (if they are in the right subject area, presented in the right format, etc.).

Role and responsibilities

The assistant editor is often responsible for managing the administration of the editorial office: ensuring the efficient flow of papers from submission to final decision, and keeping all members of the editorial team well informed.

Assistant editors are often expected to:

- assist the editor in implementing the policies of the journal;
- correspond and work with authors, editorial board members and reviewers;
- manage and maintain the manuscript tracking system;
- maintain records and produce reports of manuscripts received, accepted, rejected, etc.;
- communicate decisions to authors and deal with queries;
- ensure efficient flow of papers through the editorial office, and develop improvements in the management of papers.

> What skills do you think that an assistant editor requires? What is their job description, and what responsibilities do you think they should be expected to undertake?

Technical editors, language editors and copy editors

After a paper has been accepted, it may still require some work to ensure that it is accurate and easily readable. Some journals employ technical, language and copy editors to undertake this work. These positions may be staff or may be freelance individuals hired by the journal to undertake the work as required. Some journals include these tasks within the duties of the assistant editor(s), particularly in academic settings.

Technical editors are expected to advise on the content of the article and to review for clarity and accuracy – for example suggesting rewriting of some sections, or recommending that a figure is better represented as a table. Many journals do not employ technical editors, and rely on the reviewers and editors to provide this advice.

Language editors ensure that the language is correct and readable (i.e. understandable). For example, they may need to correct poorly expressed and grammatically incorrect text. This applies as equally to authors writing in their mother tongue as it does to text written by authors whose native language is different from the language of publication.

Copy editors are expected to ensure that the style is correct and consistent and matches the journal's style, and that the article is complete – for example that references cited in the text appear in the list of references. They also mark up the typescript ready for composition, indicating where figures should go, etc. A copy editor is also usually required to check the page proofs, to ensure that no errors have been introduced during the production processes.

There is frequently a great deal of overlap between these three roles, and many journals employ one person to undertake this work, or rely on volunteers or other members of the editorial team. In university settings, it may be possible to link up with another faculty, e.g. a language teaching faculty, to obtain support for copy/language editing.

Technical, language and copy editors are frequently not specialists in the journal discipline, but they usually have a basic understanding of the subject matter. They take responsibility for ensuring that the content of articles is presented in a consistent, readable and accurate manner. Where journals rely on their reviewers and other editors to ensure that papers are presented well, it should be noted that not only does this place additional burden on those roles, but that they may not have the attention to linguistic detail that good technical, language or copy editors have.

These editors may have to work closely with authors if an article requires a lot of clarification. It is common for queries to be identified that require answers from the authors – for example, a text citation that does not appear in the list of references, a reference that seems to be inaccurate, or clearance of a section rewritten by the technical editor. Therefore such people need good communication skills to be able to deal tactfully and directly with authors on behalf of the journal. Other journals require all queries to go through the editorial office.

In some small journals, where resources are very limited, the burden of copy editing may be placed on the authors themselves. This usually results in lower quality presentation and may not solve problems of readability, accuracy and consistency.

Role and responsibilities

The role of technical, language and copy editors is to ensure that the published articles are consistent, accurate and readable.

A set of checklists is given in Annex 4, indicating the range of tasks expected. In general, technical, language and copy editors are expected to:

- ensure that the correct structure for the corresponding section of the journal has been followed;
- improve the presentation and wording so that the text is easy to read and understand;
- develop and maintain a style sheet as a record of decisions taken concerning spelling, hyphenation, format, etc.;
- ensure correctness and consistency in the use of terms, especially technical ones;
- eliminate unnecessary and repeated material, simplify long and complicated sentences, eliminate unnecessary words;
- check that tables and figures are correctly cited in the text;
- advise on the selection and effective use of tables and illustrations;
- edit tables and figures so that they prove their point and their information ties with the text;

- check all totals and percentages;
- ensure that all cross-references are correct and that all bibliographic citations match the reference list;
- check that the references used are not grossly or overwhelmingly outdated;
- ensure that the article is complete – that it has the author addresses, email contact numbers, etc.;
- mark up the manuscript or proof with all necessary instructions for composition or printing.

What other duties would you expect a technical, language or copy editor to undertake? Does your journal require one person to undertake these roles, or do you require more than one person? Is it more suitable for you to employ a full-time person, or to use a freelance person on a contract basis?

Editorial boards and advisory boards

An editorial board is an independent body which is not directly involved with the running of the journal but which provides the editor with advice and feedback about the direction, scope and content of the journal. Depending on the journal, the board may take different forms.

In some journals the role of the board is essentially that of a body of core reviewers, who provide advice and feedback to the journal team. They will also be asked to endorse any changes that the editor may wish to introduce to the journal, and to provide information regarding changes in discipline and suggestions for future contents. Many members of editorial boards wish to support the journal by providing advice and feedback, but are either inexperienced or do not have the time to work more closely with the editor, as the associate editors do. These editorial boards tend to be large, with members from around the world. Members are usually appointed by the editor.

In some journals the role of the board is more closely concerned with governance and requires more commitment from its members. For instance, they may be required to approve new members in the editorial team, elect the chief and executive editors in consultation with the owners, perform strategic and concrete actions affecting the function of the journal, and share in making policy decisions. The board may be responsible for complying with the guidelines and procedures of their sponsoring organization, including fiscal responsibility. Board members are usually appointed by the owners upon the editor's advice.

Whether the board takes on the latter role or the former, it is usually composed of a group of highly qualified and reputed professionals, or scholars with a strong research background. It usually includes the "working" editors as well, e.g. associate editors. By joining the editorial board they endorse the journal based on the quality of the content. To ensure efficiency, the functions of the board should be clearly defined, and its members should have varied interests and expertise. The size of the board depends on the size and scope of the journal.

The term of service of a board member should be limited, in order to promote new ideas; it is common for the journal to ask people to serve for a 3-year term, which may be renewable. The board should hold periodic meetings when ideas for the structure and scope of the journal can be discussed.

Role and responsibilities

The editorial board's key role is to endorse the content of the journal, including its scope and structure. They are also expected to support the editor by providing feedback and advice as required.

The editorial board is expected to undertake some or all of the following:

- act as a source of advice and support to the editor;
- act as reviewers or suggest reviewers;
- discuss and solve any problems that might face the journal;
- contribute to the writing of editorials and invited articles;
- solicit articles for the journal;
- make policy decisions and approve the journal's by-laws;
- supervise and monitor the implementation of journal policies;
- make decisions on financial issues;
- help in decision-making when reviewers' opinions on submitted manuscripts are not in agreement;
- serve as the journal's representative to the international scientific community;
- use their professional influence to help raise the profile of the journal.

Take a look at your editorial or advisory board, and identify what roles they currently undertake. Are you making best use of your editorial board? Are there additional roles that you would like them to undertake? Do you have any gaps (in expertise or geographical representation) that you need to fill?

2.2 Authors

Objective: The editor will be able to prepare and publish clear instructions for authors, and establish effective mechanisms for communication and interaction with authors.

It is imperative that the journal maintains good relationships with authors, and the editor and the editorial office are expected to provide the following services to all contributing, or submitting, authors.

Communication with authors

All communication with authors should be fair, courteous and honest. The editor and the editorial office have a responsibility to communicate promptly with authors, and to ensure that they maintain high ethical standards – not disclosing confidential information, for example. Equally, authors are expected to behave in a similar manner with the journal, i.e. to be prompt and polite in their communications, and to ensure that they adhere to the ethical standards of the journal (for example disclosing any conflicts of interest). Obtaining feedback from authors is a good way for a journal to evaluate whether their communication routes are helpful for. This can be done through formal or informal surveys of authors. Where disputes arise, the editors have a responsibility to manage these amicably where possible, and to ensure that they have evidence for their decisions.

Key points for communication with authors

- Punctuality
- Professionalism
- Honesty
- Politeness
- Concentration on detail and clarity.

How do you evaluate your communication with authors? Do you have standard letters (or emails) for correspondence? How clear and polite are these? Are they too short, or too long?

Copyright ownership

When an author submits a manuscript to the journal they need to grant the journal the right to publish it – the act of submitting it does not confer such right to the journal. Most journals require the author to assign copyright ownership to the journal – this means that the journal literally owns the rights to copy (and publish) the article. If the author does assign copyright to the journal, then the author no longer has any rights to copy (or publish) the article elsewhere, unless the journal permits. (Many journals include a statement within their assignment form that allows the authors to use their article for "non-commercial" purposes.)

An alternative to copyright assignment is "licence to publish" in which instance the author grants the journal the exclusive rights to publish their manuscript, but they retain ownership of the article, and can use it elsewhere – perhaps in course packs for teaching. For example, the *BMJ* does not require the authors to assign copyright to them, but they require a licence to publish which grants them exclusive rights – see their online information: http://resources.bmj.com/bmj/authors/checklists-forms/licence-for-publication.

Note that whether the authors assign copyright to the journal or not, they retain moral rights in their work – this means that they must always be acknowledged as the author of the work, and the work must not be defaced in any way (for example changing the text without their approval).

It is also important to realize that in some cases the author cannot assign copyright to the journal. For example, WHO and some other institutions do not transfer copyright ownership in anything that staff (and sometimes funded researchers) have produced. Therefore even if the journal policy is to require copyright assignment to the journal, there needs to be a system in place to obtain a "licence to publish" for authors who cannot assign copyright.

Submission support

Authors must be provided with clear instructions regarding submission. This includes information on journal policy and how to comply with international standards, such as style, tables, figures, abbreviations, units of measurement, reference style and other related topics. Such instructions are traditionally published in the printed journal (usually in the first issue of the year), and must also be easy to find on the journal web site. A reference in print to the instructions on the journal web site may replace the need to print them.

A helpful guide for submissions is the *Uniform Requirements for Manuscripts Submitted to Biomedical Journals: Writing and Editing for Biomedical Publication*, which provides a great deal of information on what authors should be required to provide. The journal editors should promote this resource as the benchmark for good quality submission.

Each journal must provide up-to-date information for authors on how to submit their manuscripts, and also provide them with appropriate forms, such as declaration of authorship, copyright form, ethical clearance, etc.

Key points

- Clear guidelines for submission
- Easy submission requirements
- Helpful assistance when there are problems in submitting.

How good is your submission procedure? Take a look at the information and guidelines that you provide to your authors – are they clear, concise and polite?

Good service to authors

The journal must provide good service to authors – and this particularly includes fast and efficient manuscript processing. In particular, the time from submission to decision, and then from acceptance to publication are key to authors, and so the editorial and production office must take care to minimize delays (or "processing and publication lags") as much as possible.

Key points

- Efficient manuscript processing
- Regular communication
- Fast time from submission to decision
- Fast time from acceptance to publication.

> Do you monitor your processing and publication times? Do you set yourself targets for these times, and do you compare actual against target times? Can you identify where delays occur, and have you thought of ways to make your editorial processing more efficient?

Supporting authors

Not every author is well experienced and confident in writing articles, and journals can help them to prepare better articles. In particular, many journals provide training for authors and potential authors on scientific writing by various means, such as publishing research tips, conducting workshops, including hints and tips on writing on their web site, or direct interaction with authors. There is a wealth of information available on how to write up the results of research, and so directing authors to selected resources for self-learning may be a good way to encourage them to learn how to write and present their research. See, for example, the *BMJ* guidelines for authors: http://resources.bmj.com/bmj/authors/types-of-article/research.

Reviewers should be encouraged to provide feedback that can be given to authors to help them improve their articles, and receiving good feedback from reviewers also raises the value of the journal in the eyes of the authors.

Key points

- Helpful guides on how to write and submit
- Personal assistance and advice
- Good feedback on submitted papers.

> Do you provide your authors with help on writing articles? Can you see any immediate benefit to providing such support? What type of support could you provide?

Dealing with conflict

Unfortunately there are always likely to be some problems with authors, ranging from minor irritations to substantial conflicts. All journals must make sure that they deal with conflict in a positive manner. Examples of such problems include non-response from authors (or reviewers) beyond a given deadline, submission elsewhere after receiving reviewers' comments, dual submissions, fraud, plagiarism, pressurizing editors to speed up their decision, and not accepting a rejection. The journal should have a process for author appeals and there may be a need to appoint an independent professional (ombudsperson) to mediate in cases where there is a dispute that cannot be resolved amicably.

Key points

- Have a transparent policy/process for dealing with problems
- Do not over-react to problems
- Always attempt to resolve problems amicably.

Do you have any experience of conflicts with authors? If you do, what did you do and what did you learn?

2.3 Reviewers

Objective: The editor will be able to prepare guidelines for reviewers, develop a plan to encourage good and timely review, and develop a plan to attract new reviewers.

Reviewers are advisers to authors and editors on the quality of the manuscript. They are external experts chosen by editors to provide written opinions that allow the editor to decide whether to publish the submitted article, and provide authors with feedback that will help them to improve the manuscript. The purpose of the peer review process is to ensure the accuracy and rigour of any work prior to its being widely disseminated.

There are an increasing number of experiments to test new methods of review, and several methodologies are being tested. However, whatever methodology you use, encouraging and supporting the community of reviewers is the best way to ensure the quality of your journal content.

Communication with reviewers

It is important for all journals to build good relationships with their pool of reviewers. To this end the journal must establish good communication channels with them, including responding politely and promptly. It is also important to provide reviewers with all the information that they require, both when approaching them and when asking them to undertake a review. For example, it is generally good policy to ask if a reviewer is free to undertake a review rather than to simply send them an article, and when asking them, to give them the title and abstract of the article and the deadline for returning the review.

Depending on your reviewing methodology and the community of reviewers that you use, you may wish to share reviewer comments with other reviewers, and you may also decide to publish the reviewer comments next to the articles.

Key points

- Publish a description of the reviewing policy and process of the journal on the journal web site, and perhaps in the first printed issue of each year.
- Select competent professionals to act as reviewers for the journal, each in his/her own area of expertise. This selection should be based on sound criteria, (e.g. use may be made of the FAME tool for selecting reviewers).
- Ensure reviewers are only sent articles within their areas of expertise.
- Inform reviewers about the final decision made on manuscripts they reviewed.

Do you have standard letters for dealing with reviewers? What information do you provide them with, and is this information comprehensive but also concise?

Supporting reviewers

As with authors, it is important that the journal supports its reviewers since they are also potential authors and editorial board members. In particular, it is important to provide them with clear guidelines on what they are expected to do. You may also consider including standard forms and checklists to make it easier for them to provide useful feedback for the editors and authors. Whether you wish them to make changes and comments on a hard copy and post it back to you, or to do so online, or to email you a list of changes, it is important to make the whole process as easy as possible.

It is also important not to demand too much from reviewers – for instance requiring that they provide their review in a particular way that is excessively time-consuming for them. Equally it is important that you recognize the value that they add to the editorial process. This is done not only by thanking them privately, but also by finding ways to publicly thank them for their work. It is common for journals to include a list of reviewers in the last issue of the year, and/or provide free subscriptions to key reviewers, or perhaps free copies of the journal. Some journals name the reviewers at the end of the published article (where blind reviewing is not used).

In order to provide authors with helpful feedback for improving their manuscripts, you ideally want to be able to send them feedback directly from the reviewers. To allow you to do this you must make sure that the feedback is helpful, positive and politely written. Therefore it is important to ensure that your reviewers are aware that some of their comments will be sent directly to the authors, and you may wish to emphasize the need to be constructive in their criticisms of the papers. You may be able to provide training workshops, or at least guidelines, to help instruct reviewers in the following communication skills: punctuality, sincerity, professionalism, responsibility, honesty, politeness, use of argument in disputes and concentration on detail and clarity.

Key points

- Avoid overworking busy reviewers – for example, sending them manuscripts too frequently.
- Supply reviewers with the journal guidelines and expectations for reviewing manuscripts.
- Request reviewers to be critical but constructive and courteous.
- Reward reviewers with incentives such as free subscriptions, free copies, and recognition of their contribution.

What support could you provide to reviewers to help them with their work? How can you reward reviewers who work for you?

Dealing with conflict

As with authors, it is important for the journal to have clear guidelines to avoid conflicts when articles are reviewed. Within reviewing, the most common problem is that of competing interests (also called conflict of interest). This happens most frequently when a reviewer has been sent a paper in the same area that they are researching.

Remember that the reviewers only advise the editors, and there is always the opportunity to have the paper reviewed by another person if you suspect that there may be bias in the review you have received.

Key points

- Ask reviewers to disclose to the editor any potential competing interests with the paper under review.
- Ask reviewers to respect and maintain the confidentiality of the contents of the manuscript and not to disclose it to anyone without the consent of the editor.
- Ask reviewers not to make use of, or quote from, the manuscripts they are reviewing before they are published.
- Ask reviewers to obtain written consent of the editor if, for any reason, they want to refer the manuscript to another colleague.
- Ask reviewers not to contact the author regarding the manuscript without consulting the editor.
- Send manuscripts to at least one foreign or external reviewer when working for a journal that serves a small scientific community, in order to avoid competing interests.

What can you do to minimize the problem of competing interests in reviewers? Do you have a system to easily identify where there may be a problem?

2.4 Readers

Objective: The editor will be able to develop a plan to enhance readership of the journal and encourage feedback from readers.

It can be easy to forget about readers, as the priority of most editors is to find good quality articles to publish. However it can be argued that readers are the main reason for any journal to exist, and it is important to remember that this community is as important as any other.

In particular, the journal must identify exactly what their target readers want (their needs and interests), and ensure that at all times they provide their readership with the quality of publication that they require. This means ensuring that the content is appropriate for the readership both in the way it is presented, and the type of articles that the journal publishes. Journal editors must be familiar with best practice in editing, peer review, research ethics, methods of investigation, and the rationale and evidence base supporting them, and ensure that they clearly identify the different type of content (research articles and opinions, for example). To gain and retain trust of the readership the journal must be transparent in its processes (for example what type of peer review it undertakes), who funds the journal (as this may bias its operation), and be willing to admit mistakes – publishing errata and corrections if required.

Part of the responsibility of a journal is to ensure, wherever possible, continued access to their publication, and particularly in the online environment it is vital to ensure that archiving solutions are in place so that even if a journal discontinues its publication, readers can access the old issues. This can be undertaken by negotiating archival agreements with national libraries or international bodies, such as PubMed Central in the USA (http://www.pubmedcentral.nih.gov/).

Obtaining feedback from readers is important for journal development, and this can be implemented by encouraging letters to be submitted, or undertaking readership surveys. Within the online environment there may be an opportunity to engage the community using Web 2.0 tools such as discussion forums.

Key points

- Independence: Editorial decisions must be based on the validity of the work and its importance to readers, and not the policies or commercial successes of the owners or the self-interest of the editors.
- Transparency: There must be transparency in regard to the ownership and funding of the journal, authorship and research within the journal.
- Access: Content should be delivered in appropriate formats, and suitable distribution channels put in place, to ensure the target audience is reached.
- Longevity: The journal must ensure continued access to, and long-term preservation of, its published information.
- Communication: The editor should encourage feedback, for example through letters to the editor and readership surveys.
- Transparency: The journal must publish corrections, retractions and critiques of published articles where required.

What do you feel you could learn from your readers? Have you ever undertaken a readership survey? Do you feel confident that you know what your readers value and read in your journal? Do you encourage feedback from your readers, and if you do not, how would you encourage this?

2.5 Publishers, owners or sponsoring society

Objective: The editor will be able to clarify and develop strong working relationships with the publishers, owners or sponsors of the journal.

The publisher, owner or sponsoring society or association is an important member of the overall journal team, and there should be a professional and trusting relationship between it and the editorial team. In particular, the different roles must be clarified and honoured, particularly with respect to editorial freedom (see Section 1).

Equally, the editor has a responsibility to the publisher or owner of the journal, and must ensure that s/he does not make any decisions which might adversely affect the business of the owner or publisher without informing them. It is likely that the owner or publisher will select the printers and other companies supplying publishing services, and the editor must work with them on a professional basis. Where the editor selects people or companies with whom to work s/he must do so on the basis of merit and cost, and be able to explain and justify the choice to the owner of the journal if required.

The editor is also responsible for maintaining records and reporting to the journal owner, usually on an annual basis, and these reports should always be honest and comprehensive. In addition to reporting on the journal's activities, editors should inform the owner or sponsoring organization of any misconduct detected and resolved during the year, and of any changes to editorial structure. They must also keep the owner or sponsoring organization informed of any changes to their activities that might affect their editorial role, e.g. becoming employed by a pharmaceutical company.

Key points

- The editor should report to the highest governing body of the owning organization.
- The editor should ensure that his/her work is above reproach.

Do you have a clear working relationship with your publisher, owner or funding association? Do you feel that there are any conflicts, and if you do, what can you do to resolve them? Do you provide them with regular information about the journal, and what type of information do they find most valuable?

Resources and further reading

COPE. *Best practice guidelines for journal editors.* UK, Committee on Publication Ethics (COPE), 2002. Visited 29 June 2009. http://publicationethics.org/code-conduct

CSE. *Editorial policy statements approved by the Council of Science Editors Board of Directors.* [undated] USA, Council of Science Editors (CSE). Visited 29 June 2009. http://www.councilscienceeditors.org/services/draft_approved.cfm

FAME. *FAME guidelines for selecting reviewers.* Kenya, Forum for African Medical Editors (FAME), 2005. Visited 29 June 2009. http://apps.who.int/tdr/svc/resources/partnerships-networks/fame-guidelines

FAME. *FAME guidelines on improving the quality of submissions.* Kenya, Forum for African Medical Editors (FAME), 2005. Visited 29 June 2009. http://apps.who.int/tdr/svc/resources/partnerships-networks/fame-guidelines

Hames I. Editorial boards: realizing their potential. *Learned publishing.* 2001, 14: 247-256.

ICMJE. *Uniform requirements for manuscripts submitted to biomedical journals: writing and editing for biomedical publication.* Updated October 2008. International Committee of Medical Journal Editors (ICMJE). Visited 29 June 2009. http://www.icmje.org

Utiger RD. *Syllabus for prospective and newly appointed editors.* USA, World Association of Medical Editors (WAME), 2001. Visited 29 June 2009. http://www.wame.org/syllabus.htm

Marcovitch H, Williamson A. Editorial Boards. In: Maisonneuve J et al. (eds). *Science editors' handbook.* UK, European Association of Science Editors (EASE), 2007. Section 1-1.3.

Pearson CH et al. Associate editor's role in helping authors and upholding journal standards. *Agronomy Journal,* 2006, 98: 417–422. DOI: 10.2134/agronj2005.0296

Ray JG. Judging the judges: the role of journal editors. *Quarterly Journal of Medicine,* 2002, 95: 769-774.

WAME. *WAME editorial policy committee. Policy statements.* [Undated] World Association of Medical Editors (WAME), USA. Visited 29 June 2009. http://www.wame.org/wamestmt.htm

3. Product

Purpose: To enable editors to establish and maintain an effective process for producing a quality publication.

3.1 Production process

Objective: The editor will be able to establish an efficient system for production of the journal.

3.2 Quality

Objective: The editor will be able to put in place systems for quality assurance and control.

3.1 Production process

Objective: The editor will be able to establish an efficient system for production of the journal.

This section addresses the production processes required to produce the finished journal issue. It does not consider the policy decisions concerned (e.g. the criteria on which articles are accepted, or the decision to publish in print or online), which have been covered in Section 1. The steps involved in producing a journal are outlined in Figure 1.

Keeping track

A system for recording papers from submission to publication is necessary so that you can effectively manage the journal operation. If the journal is using a manuscript submission or peer review management and publishing system (e.g. Bench-press, Open Journal Systems) the tracking will be built in and take a manuscript from submission to publication, incorporating all the processes in between (reviewing, revision, editing, layout, proofing). Otherwise some kind of system is needed, which can be a simple Excel sheet, or a more complicated database.

The items that you should record include:

- the relevant details of a paper – e.g. title, authors, date of receipt/acceptance, type of paper (e.g. original research, review, etc.), the issue it is assigned to;
- the different stages of production, and the progress along these stages, including editing, queries to authors, layout, proofs, printing and final publication (or posting the e-version online).

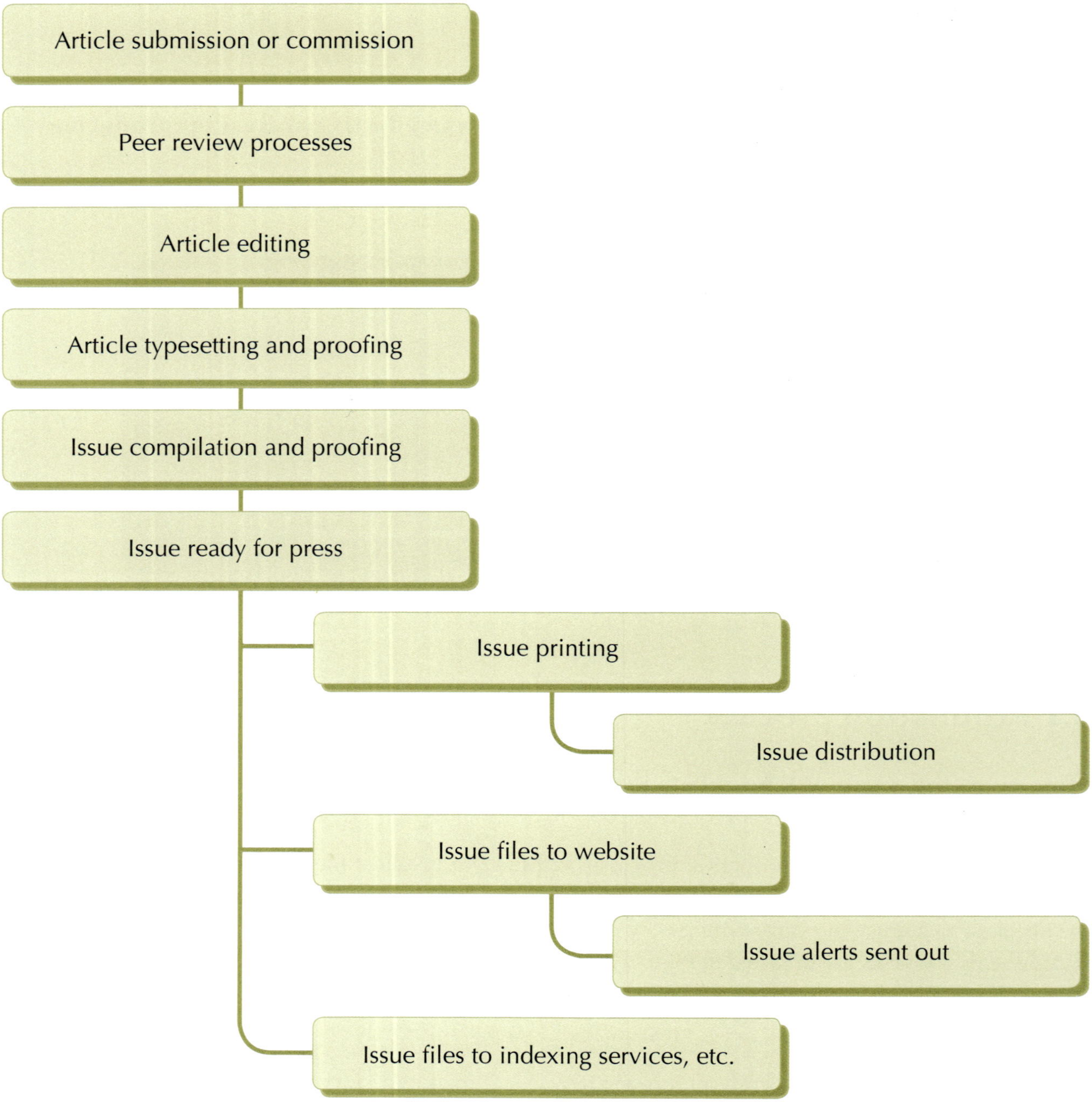

Figure 1. Steps involved in producing a journal

Scheduling

To ensure issues are published on time, a schedule is essential for the production of each issue. This should itemize each step in production and the time available for the step. It is usual for a schedule to only list the steps from "selection of articles for issue" onwards. A simplified example schedule for a quarterly journal is given in Table 1.

Table 1. Schedule for a quarterly journal

Schedule step	Time required	Dates			
		Issue 1	Issue 2	Issue 3	Issue 4
Issue selection	Day 1	25-Jan	16-Feb	18-May	17-Aug
Issue instructions to printer/typesetter	3 days	28-Jan	09-Mar	08-Jun	07-Sep
Issue proof to editor and authors for correction	4 days	01-Feb	30-Mar	29-Jun	28-Sep
Issue corrected proof to printer/typesetter	5 days	06-Feb	20-Apr	20-Jul	19-Oct
Final issue approved for press	3 days	09-Feb	11-May	10-Aug	09-Nov
E-files uploaded on website	5 days	14-Feb	16-May	15-Aug	14-Nov
Printed copies delivered ready for dispatch	21 days	02-Mar	01-Jun	31-Aug	30-Nov

The printed copy of an issue should arrive with the subscriber within the month on the cover – e.g. a March issue will arrive in March. This means that you should aim to publish the March issue at the end of February or right at the beginning of March.

Do you have an annual schedule for your journal? Are there any items not included above that should be included in your schedule (e.g. receipt of advertising material)?

Most journals operate what is called a "flow" production system. In this, each paper is set into the journal style (design) as soon as it has been accepted. It is then sent to the authors as a proof for them to check. When the articles are returned they are then "held for press". This means that they wait until the scheduled "Issue selection" date, at which time they are selected for inclusion in the journal issue.

The alternative is to operate a "batch" production system. In this, each paper that is accepted is held until the issue selection date, at which time they are all typeset, then proofed to the authors, corrected and sent to the printer, etc., in one batch.

Although the "batch" system appears to be much simpler, it is not so efficient, and can lead to issue delays. The reasons for this are as follows.

- If an author delays returning their proof, this can hold up the entire issue.
- If corrections change the pagination of an article (making it longer or shorter) this can require extensive corrections to the rest of the issue.
- If there are queries which result in a paper being de-selected, this can lead to problems filling in the space or publishing of a short issue.

Because of these possible problems, the "flow" system is usually preferred.

Editing

Even though a paper may have been reviewed in-house and peer reviewed, it is unlikely to be fit for publication and it is not until the editing stage that many technical problems and shortcomings of a paper come to light. Therefore some degree of editing is always required. The extent of editing and who does it will depend on the resources of the journal. Small journals with few resources often require the editor or perhaps members of the editorial board to undertake this. If this is the case with your journal, you need to bear in mind that most of the editorial board are volunteers with their own heavy workload – and they may not have the ideal skills to edit a paper to ensure it complies with the journal house style. It is always worth trying to secure funding for this type of editor (whether in-house or freelance).

Post-acceptance editing can be divided into three types with the same person responsible for all three types, or different people for each (see Section 2 for more information).

- Mechanical editing: in which the manuscript is checked for completeness (all pages, authors' names, affiliations, tables and figures are present). This could be done by a secretary according to a checklist and is essential as it is easy for some components to go missing.
- Copy editing: in which the paper is edited for grammar, spelling, suitability of tables/figures for publication, correctness of references and conformity of the paper with the house style. It may also include insertion of mark-up in preparation for layout. This requires someone with a good command of the language of the paper and familiarity with the journal style and mark-up tags. Copy editing can of course include mechanical editing.
- Technical editing: in which the paper is substantially edited for conciseness, clarity, accuracy and consistency and will probably result in queries being sent to the authors. This requires someone with both a good command of the language of the paper and knowledge of scientific research and research writing. Technical editing can include copy editing and mechanical editing.

Editing can be done on-screen or on hard copy, depending on how the journal is set up and who is doing the editing. Professional editors will work on-screen which can streamline the production processes (avoiding postage, and making it quicker for the printer/typesetter to undertake the layout). Generally on-screen editing is most easily done in a word processing program such as Word but it is sometimes done in the desk-top publishing (DTP) application itself (e.g. PageMaker, InDesign, Quark).

In your own journal, who edits the papers once they have been accepted? What process do you have for undertaking this work, and for speaking to the authors if there are any queries?

Page layout and proofing

After the papers have been edited, they will be put into page layout (sent for composition). When this has been done the proofs must be sent to the authors for checking. The reason for this is so that they can ensure there have been no errors in converting the electronic files they sent and, if you have had to re-type any content, no errors have been introduced.

Who should undertake the composition? Can you do it in-house with a desk-top publishing application, or do you have the funds (and is it more efficient) to pay a freelance person (or company) or the printer (if they have the facilities) – to do this work? This decision is affected by the type of content as well as the funding available, and the type of e-publishing that you undertake.

When you publish both online and in print, it is possible that you will have two layouts – one for the print version, plus HTML for the online version. Where a journal produces two formats it is usual that the most complex (usually the print layout) is undertaken first, and it is this version that is supplied to the author for checking. Only after this version has been corrected and approved is the HTML version prepared. This is often a simple matter of conversion and need only be checked in-house for conversion quality.

Proofs are now usually supplied to the authors as PDF files to save the time and expense of posting paper copies. However, most authors will then print out their proofs, annotate them and post, fax or scan and email them back to the journal within a specific time-frame (which may be as little as 72 hours). If they have the correct software (e.g. Adobe Acrobat 9.0) they can annotate on the PDF file directly and return this electronically, but many authors do not have this facility (and they would have to purchase it) so a journal cannot insist that they do this.

If you are using an online journal management system (e.g. Open Journal Systems), then this will provide tools to alert authors when their proof is ready, and to remind them when it is expected back. If you do not have such a system, then you will need an alternative system to send proofs out, chase their return, and monitor their status.

You should always expect some corrections at the proof stage. Sometimes there are outstanding queries from the manuscript which the author has to answer on the proof. Other times there are some mistakes in the layout, and sometimes the author wishes to change some of the text. Ideally you should always aim for minimum corrections at proof – and if you have a good editing system in place this will help to minimize proof corrections.

Some publishers only ask the authors to check the proofs, but it is advisable for the journal to also check them. This can be done by the editorial staff, or by a freelance person. Commonly the editorial staff responsible for this work will check the proofs that the author has returned, so they can look at any changes that the author requests (as the author may be incorrect in asking for some changes), as well as checking for stylistic correctness (i.e. that the layout is correct, and that the article contains all the required content – figures, references, etc.).

What system do you have for providing proofs to authors, and ensuring that they return them on time? Can it be improved?

Compiling the issue

Issue selection

When the time has come to compile the issue, the following actions need to be undertaken:

- determining the order of the papers (and which papers to include within the issue – you may decide to hold some over to the next issue);

- writing an editorial, or "highlights of the issue", if you include such content;
- selecting notices, news items, advertisements, fillers, corrigenda, etc., if you include such content;
- preparing the table of contents, and updating the cover.

This work is generally undertaken by the editor with the assistance of the editorial office staff.

What items do you need to consider when selecting and preparing an issue? How efficient are your methods for undertaking this operation, and can you think of one area that could be improved?

Issue layout and proofing

Once the selection has been made, the issue layout needs to be finalized. With a "flow" system this will require final correction of each paper, typesetting of any additional content, inclusion of any advertising artwork, etc., and pagination of the entire issue.

When the issue layout has been finalized, it should also be proofed. At this time only the new content needs to be read carefully, but the layout and pagination needs to be carefully checked.

It is usual that the editor will always see a proof of the final issue, so they can authorize publication. However they may not be expected to do the final checking of corrections, etc. Their role is to authorize the content – not only the selection of articles, but also any advertising, etc.

Issue printing

When an issue has been compiled, typeset and proofed, it is ready for printing and publishing online. At this point the electronic files need to be supplied to the printer, and to whoever manages the web site.

It is usual to contract a printer for the year – i.e. to print every issue during that year – and to agree a schedule with them. This avoids problems in funding and agreeing terms for each issue, and ensuring consistency of printing throughout the year. When you make an agreement with your printer it is important to discuss and agree the delivery details. Printers have different preferences for file types and how they are prepared, and it is important to discuss this with them when you first agree to use them. If you change any of the software that is used to prepare the issue for press, you must also alert them, as this may introduce problems when they receive the files.

You also need to agree on how they deliver the printed copies. Some printers will post out to your subscribers (or association members), but require you to provide labels. You should agree how they deliver the printed copies: if they are posting out, then what type of envelope they use; if they are delivering the bulk to you, then what size pallets they will use, and whether you require them to put the journals into boxes, or leave them loose on the pallet.

It is recommended that you ask the printer to provide you with a proof to approve before they print and bind all the copies. This is to ensure that there are no problems when they import your electronic files. When you have been working with a printer for a long time, and experience no problems, you may be able to forego this stage (which could save you money and time).

Some publishers provide their authors with a small quantity of their articles printed and stapled (sometimes with a cover), which the authors can use for promotional purposes. This is becoming less common, and journals often supply the authors with a PDF of their final article instead of an offprint. If you supply either print or PDF offprints to the authors, you must remember to implement a system to produce these efficiently.

Some journals offer their authors the opportunity to purchase additional offprints, and also offer these for sale to other companies, such as pharmaceutical companies. Depending on the type of journal, these can be a valuable source of income. If you undertake this, then you need to ensure that you have a system to manage the ordering and delivery of such offprints, as well as management of the billing and income for such work.

It is good practice to send the printer a print order for every issue. On this order you should include the following items:

- journal title and issue;
- number of pages, and special instructions (e.g. if one part is to be printed in colour);
- quantity to print (although this is usually agreed at the start of the year, you may wish to change it);
- quantity of offprints (if required);
- required delivery date.

Are you happy with the printing service that you receive (not only the quality of print, but the timekeeping and customer service)? Can you think of any improvements you could make to the way in which you work with your printer?

Online issue publication

Some journals are published online only, and others are published both online and in print. If you publish online only, then the processes for issue publication are very similar to those for a "traditional" journal, since you still need to edit each article, and will want the authors to check their articles before they go "live" on the journal web site. If you publish article-by-article (i.e. not grouped in issues), then there is no issue selection process to be undertaken, and so the production processes are very much simplified. If, however, you do group by issue, then the issue compilation processes are similar to those in a print journal. If you publish in print and online, you may have different content for each version, in which case you need to build in procedures during the issue compilation stages to allow for preparation of the separate issues (print and online).

For an online journal, you need to supply appropriate files for the online publication to whoever uploads them and maintains your web site, in the same way that you arrange for files to be supplied to the printer. If you publish online as PDF articles, you will need to prepare the table of contents with links to the relevant PDF. Remember that the PDF used to publish online differs from that used to print (smaller file size for quicker downloading). If you generate PDFs for your printers, these will be a high-resolution file; however they will be too big for online publishing (for which you need a low-resolution file). You should seek advice to determine the best way of publishing online, and this will be – in part – determined by the funding that you have available.

Online hosting of your journal should also be carefully considered. There are two options: to host the journal on your own institutional web site or to join an aggregating service. To host on your own web site may be cheaper, however your IT staff may not have the specialist skills and knowledge to ensure that you have a highly visible service able to provide the type of user features which are increasingly demanded by authors, readers and librarians. Aggregating services (such as IngentaConnect, HighWire and Atypon) provide high quality services and valuable advice for journals, but they can be quite expensive. If you decide to host the journal on your own web site the open source software "Open Journal Systems" can provide suitable publishing software which integrates with an online manuscript submission and tracking system (discussed above).

If you publish online, do you think your procedures are efficient? How do you present your content online? Look at other journals that you like and see if there are things they do which you could emulate.

3.2 Quality

Objective: The editor will be able to put in place systems for quality assurance and control.

Principles

The issue of quality arises at the outset of a journal. A fundamental issue is the budget available. A generous budget is a distinct advantage although this does not mean you cannot produce a quality journal on a limited budget – it is just harder. Conversely a large budget does not guarantee a quality journal. In this respect it is important to have a clear vision for the journal and its scope. Don't be over-ambitious; a few good papers published every three months on time is better than a monthly journal with papers of poor or erratic quality published late. While greater periodicity may be a goal, it should not be at the expense of quality.

The quality of a journal is only as good as the quality of the papers it publishes. No amount of detailed editing, professional layout, timely production, good design and superior printing will disguise poor content. To use valuable editing and layout skills and time on poor quality papers is a waste. However, if a paper is fundamentally sound but perhaps has shortcomings linguistically, or in reporting and presentation, then the time spent on polishing the paper (the review and editing stages especially) is well worthwhile. It is worth remembering that many researchers may be preparing papers in a language that is not their mother tongue, which can affect the presentation of the paper. Acceptance of an article should therefore be dependent on the science and not on the quality of the language.

The issue of ensuring the quality of papers submitted and accepted is dealt with in the earlier sections. Here we focus on the issue of the quality of the product assuming the content meets the required standards. It is difficult to over-emphasize the importance of quality. No matter how small and limited the journal is, if it maintains a good quality in terms of content, design and periodicity, this will contribute significantly to attracting notice which can lead to an upward spiral of greater visibility, better papers being submitted, indexing in the international indexing systems, etc. To produce a poor quality journal with erratic publication will lead to a downward spiral of less interest, poorer papers and possibly eventual closure.

Where do you feel that your journal adds quality to the scholarly communication cycle?

Key quality issues

Vision

A clear vision for the journal and its scope is needed (see Section 1.1). Without this vision, quality will be hard to maintain.

Budget

A guaranteed adequate budget to ensure that the journal can be maintained is needed. Why start a journal that can only be sustained for a few issues? The budget will have a fundamental impact on the journal and will dictate to a great extent the services that can be afforded. Within the constraints of the budget you need to ensure the best quality possible.

Quality issues that need to be considered within the context of the budget are:

- review process – although this is generally done on a voluntary basis, there are certain costs involved to manage the process;
- editing – this can be undertaken by volunteer staff or by external companies, depending on available skills and budget;
- design and layout – can also be done by volunteers, by in-house staff or by external contractors, depending on the available budget;
- printing, including: type/weight of paper; colour or black and white printing, cover design and colour; binding and finishing;
- print run and periodicity;
- distribution and circulation costs.

Peer review quality

The quality of peer review is determined by the reviewers and the manner in which the process is managed. The journal can add quality to the process by managing it efficiently, selecting good reviewers, and providing support to the reviewers to help them provide good reviews quickly. For example, the journal should provide clear guidance on what it is seeking to publish, and how to prepare reviews for the journal. The journal should also maintain records of reviewers, so they know who to select for different papers and the selection process is optimized.

> What value do you add to the peer review process by your own internal processes?

Timely and regular production and dissemination

A journal that does not publish regularly, and on the dates that it promises, will quickly be regarded as a poor quality publication. It is important to both readers and authors that material is published quickly and regularly. This is also a prerequisite for any indexing and abstracting institution, such as Index Medicus. Therefore, establishing a publication schedule, and keeping to it are as important as being seen to process and publish individual articles quickly. Many journals now include the date of acceptance on each article so that readers (and potential authors) can see how quickly articles are published.

> Do you publish on time? What are your average submission-to-acceptance, and your acceptance-to-publication times? Can you improve on them?

Design

It is important to present the journal content in a way that is professional and appealing to the readers. Designs do not need to be complex, but it is important that the journal establishes a style which makes its content easily readable, and that it is consistent in the way that it presents its content. Colour is – mistakenly – often used as a measure of quality, but there is no necessity to publish in colour unless the type of photographs or other illustrations require this. Of more importance is how easy it is for readers to find the content, either in print or online (e.g. individual articles, cited references, etc.), and how easy it is to read.

As the design of the journal will not be frequently changed, it is worthwhile spending both time and money at the outset to come up with an effective and attractive design. If you decide to change the design at any time, this should be implemented at the beginning of a volume to preserve identity.

> Look at other journals that you like, see what designs they use. Do you think the design of your journal is good enough, or does it require some re-thinking?

Communication

Good and timely communication with (and between) all the stakeholders in journal publishing (e.g. authors, printers, etc.) is important. It is worth taking time to set up good and speedy communication lines between all those involved who need to interact and to ensure that the journal responds promptly to enquiries.

Systems

There are both technological and practical systems that all journals should ensure they have in place if they are to add quality to the scholarly communication system. Practical systems refer to actual processes – knowing who should do which action, how long it should take them, etc. Technological systems mean using technology to the maximum effect to help you become more efficient.

Systems that will help ensure the quality of the product include the following:

- Tracking system: to ensure appropriate, smooth and timely flow of material from receipt to editorial decision to publication. This may involve a database, an Excel workbook, or some other filing system. Ensuring that it is kept up-to-date is important, as is making use of the information captured to improve quality, e.g. by finding the average time it takes to peer review articles.
- Peer review system: to ensure constructive and prompt evaluation of manuscripts (see Section 1). This involves selecting reviewers, sending invitations, chasing late reviews, etc. Technological systems may help in the selection and monitoring of reviewers (creation of automatic reminders), and help in online submission of reviews.
- Editing and proofing system: to ensure all material for publication is presented to the highest standard and conforms with the house style (see also the checklists in Annex 4).
- Production and distribution system: to ensure timely and wide distribution of the journal as soon as it is published, in a format that readers can access and read easily.

> How do you use technology in your different systems? Are there opportunities for streamlining some of your systems to make the journal more efficient and of higher quality?

Resources and further reading

Standards and style. In: Maisonneuve J et al. (eds). *Science editors' handbook.* UK, European Association of Science Editors (EASE), 2007. Part 2.

Publishing and printing. In: Maisonneuve J et al. (eds). *Science editors' handbook.* UK, European Association of Science Editors (EASE), 2007. Part 4.

Open Journal Systems. Visited 29 June 2009. http://pkp.sfu.ca/?q=ojs

Page G, Campbell R, Meadows J. *Journal publishing.* Cambridge, UK, Cambridge University Press, 1997.

Tananbaum G, Holmes L. The evolution of Web-based peer-review systems. *Learned Publishing,* 2008, 21:300-306. DOI: 10.1087/095315108X356734

Annex 1. SWOT analysis

SWOT = Strengths, Weaknesses, Opportunities, Threats

Undertaking an analysis of the journal's strengths and weaknesses is a useful way to identify what the journal is good at, and can build on, and what it is not good at, and needs to address. Identifying opportunities and threats (which relate to the "external environment" that affect the journal) can help you to develop the journal and ensure that it operates successfully in a complex economic and academic environment .

Strengths include items such as:

- good editors;
- fast manuscript processing times;
- clear aims and scope.

Weaknesses include items such as:

- too few reviewers;
- slow manuscript processing times;
- too few submissions.

Opportunities include items such as:

- new "hot topics" in your discipline;
- online publishing;
- changes in government policy.

Threats include items such as:

- competitor journals;
- expensive technologies;
- decreasing library budgets.

How to undertake a SWOT analysis

There are no fixed rules: the editor can do this alone, or ask members of the publishing team to each undertake the analysis (which might be an interesting way to obtain different views). The purpose of undertaking the analysis is to use the findings to prioritize what issues and items the journal should address in order to become more successful.

Strengths	Weaknesses
• *Author demand*	• *Poor quality of papers*
Opportunities	**Threats**
• *No competition*	• *Institutional changes may affect funding*

Annex 2. Indexing services

Note: This list contains a selection only and is not exhaustive.

African Index Medicus (**WHO**)
African health literature and information sources
http://indexmedicus.afro.who.int/

BIOSIS
Biological Abstracts
http://thomsonreuters.com/products_services/science/science_products/life_sciences/biology/biosis

CAB Abstracts
Applied life sciences
http://www.cabi.org/datapage.asp?iDocID=165

CEHAART (**WHO**)
Environmental health articles database
http://www.emro.who.int/Library/Databases/wxis.exe/Library/Databases/iah/?IsisScript=iah/iah.xic&base=cehaart&lang=i

CAB Global Health
Public health research and practice
http://www.cabi.org/datapage.asp?iDocID=169

CSA (**Cambridge Scientific Abstracts**)
Biological sciences
http://www.csa.com/factsheets/biolclust-set-c.php

Chemical Abstracts
Chemistry and related sciences
http://info.cas.org/

CSA Neurosciences Abstracts
Vertebrate and invertebrate neuroscience, emphasizing basic research
http://www.csa.com/factsheets/neurosciences-set-c.php

CINAHL
Cumulative Index to Nursing and Allied Health Literature
http://www.ebscohost.com/cinahl/

Current contents
Includes sections on clinical medicine, life sciences, and behavioural sciences
http://www.thomsonreuters.com/products_services/science/science_products/scholarly_research_analysis/research_discovery/current_contents?parentKey=433717

EMBASE
Biomedical and pharmacological bibliographic database
http://www.info.embase.com/about/coverage.shtml

EMRMEDEX
Biomedical journals published in Eastern Mediterranean Region
http://www.emrmedex.com/list.asp

Index Medicus for the Eastern Mediterranean Region (IMEMR) (WHO)
Health and health-related literature in the WHO Eastern Mediterranean Region
http://www.emro.who.int/LIN/imemr.htm

International Pharmaceutical Abstracts (IPA)
Pharmaceutical science and health related literature
http://www.csa.com/factsheets/supplements/ipa.php

ISI Web of Science
Broad database covering different specialties – note that the database also produces the Journal Citation Reports (JCR) which allocate impact factors
http://scientific.thomson.com/mjl/selection/

PubMed and MEDLINE
Biomedical journal literature
http://www.nlm.nih.gov/pubs/factsheets/pubmed.html

PSYCINFO
Psychological literature
http://www.apa.org/psycinfo/

SCOPUS
Broad database covering different specialties
http://www.info.scopus.com/

Zoological Record
Animal biology
http://science.thomsonreuters.com/training/zr/

Annex 3. Sample manuscript flow chart

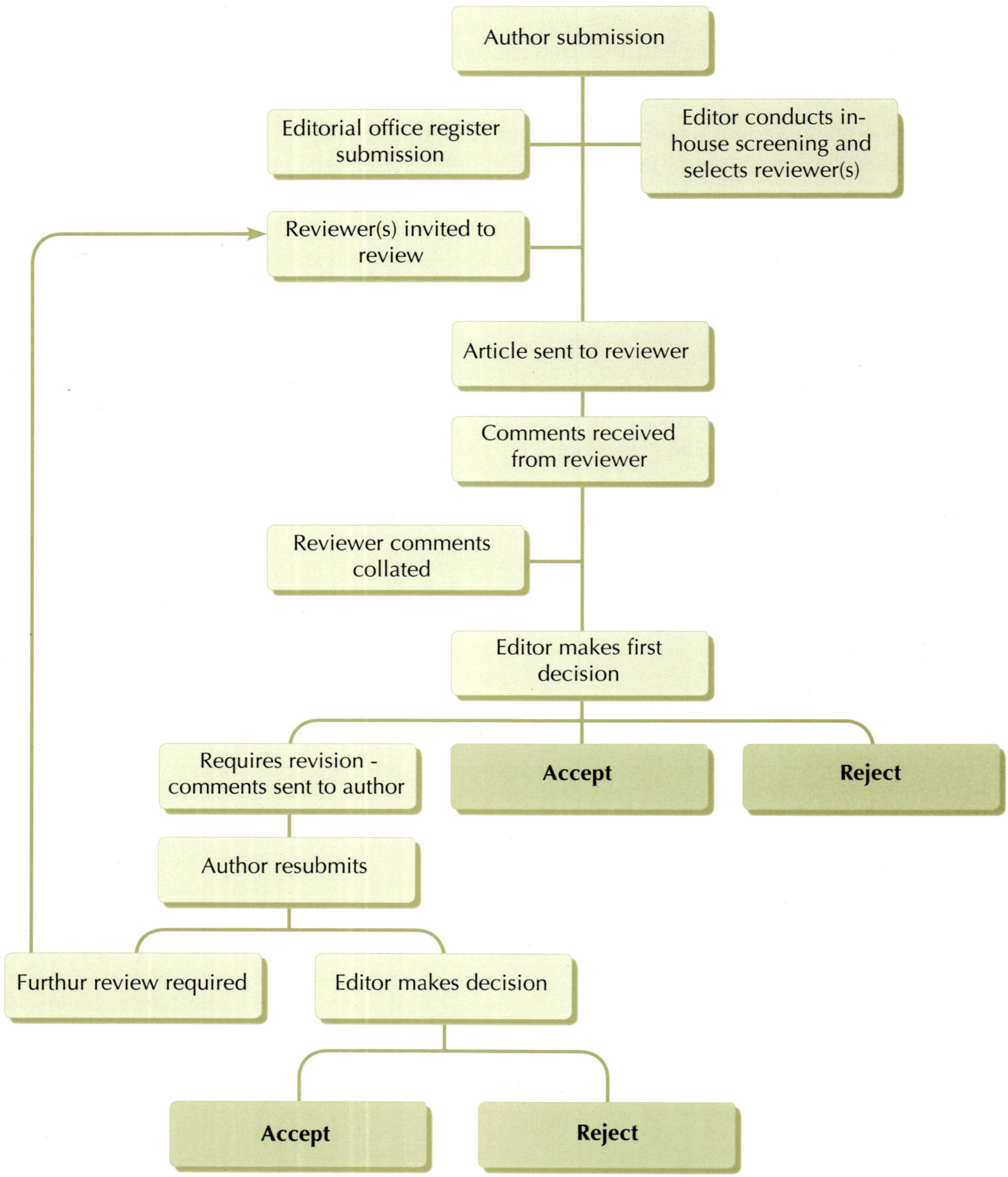

Annex 4. Checklists

Mechanical editing

- Ensure the manuscript is complete: all pages, figures and tables are included and required house style has been followed.
- Check the title page includes all necessary information (article title, authors' names and affiliations in full and linked, address for correspondence).
- Check the abstract is of the correct length and key words listed.

Copy editing

- Check the format of headings and paragraphs is correct and appropriate.
- Ensure the grammar, spellings and punctuation are correct and consistent with house style.
- Check the abbreviations included are appropriate and are spelled out the first time they are used.
- Ensure the use of italics, bold and quotes is appropriate and not excessive.
- Ensure units are included where necessary and used correctly (e.g. SI units).
- Check figures and tables referred to in the text are in correct numerical order.
- Check that the number of tables/figures is not excessive and comparable to the length of the paper.
- Check that tables have clear titles and column headings.
- Ensure that all abbreviations in tables are explained in the legend.
- Ensure that drawings and photographs are clear and of good quality and the caption agrees with what the figure shows.
- Check that all references in the text are also included in the reference list in the correct order, and all those in the reference list are mentioned in the text.
- Ensure that all references are in the correct format in line with journal style.
- Mark up the text ready for layout (indicate where figures, tables, etc., are to appear in the text, add journal information as required).

Technical editing

General

- Edit for conciseness and clarity of text (eliminate repetition and unnecessary text, ensure good grammar, simplify language, avoid pomposity/verbosity).
- Edit for accuracy (check errors of fact, ensure specific statements are backed up with relevant references, check numbers/percentages, additions, cross references with tables/text/abstracts, references).
- Edit for consistency – layout/check correct level of headings/check appropriate text under each heading (IMRAD).
- Edit tables/figures for accuracy and ease of reading/understanding.
- Ensure correct units are used where necessary and that they are the correct ones (preferably SI units).
- Apply house style.
- Compile queries for authors.

Title

- Does it indicate what the article is about?
- Is it clear, concise and precise?
- Is it within the word limit specified by the journal (10–12 words is a reasonable limit)?
- Is it simple and without abbreviations, jargon, excessive adjectives, strings of nouns?

Abstract

- Is it within word limit specified by the journal and in the format specified by the journal (unstructured, structured)?
- Does it say:
  - Why the study was done.
  - What the study question was
  - What was done and how. Methods used.
  - What was found. Synopsis of results including size of study groups and basic figures.
  - What the findings mean. What can be learnt?
- Do the data match what is in the text/tables?

Introduction

- Does it give background information on the study and place in context?
- Is the study justified (why was it important to conduct the study and what will it add to the body of knowledge)?
- Are the aims of the study clearly stated?

Methods (depending on the type of study)

- Is the study design indicated (cohort, cross-sectional case–control, etc.)?
- Are the time and place of the study given?
- Is the way in which participants were recruited and chosen described?
- Are inclusion/exclusion criteria adequately described?
- Are refusals to participate (and how they were dealt with) mentioned, and their effect on the study discussed? Are losses to follow-up and how they were dealt with mentioned and their effect on the study discussed?
- Are all relevant characteristics of participants described?
- Are informed consent procedures and other ethical features described?
- If a questionnaire was used, is it adequately described?
- Are the methods or experimental procedures and instruments used adequately described and referenced if necessary? Are the reasons for using a new method given and its possible limitations?
- Are genus, species and strain of animals, plants, etc., given?
- Are drug dosages/form of treatment/and how solutions were prepared with precise concentrations given?
- Are end points/outcomes defined?
- Is sample size justified?
- Are generic names used and proprietary preparation only given if relevant?
- Are details of statistical methods used adequately described, including software (version)? Is the value of statistical significance reported?
- Can the study be replicated from the details provided?

Results

- Are the results presented in a logical sequence?
- Are all relevant results reported?
- Does the text draw attention to the most significant aspects of the results?
- Are numbers reported to an appropriate degree of accuracy?
- Are P values reported appropriately?
- Are confidence intervals given?

Table/figures

- Are all tables, figures and other illustrations referred to in the text and numbered in the order in which they are first referred to?
- Are data in tables/figure the same as in the text and abstract?
- Are all the figures/tables useful, necessary and effective?
- Do the tables/figures make complete sense on their own without reference to the text?
- If a table is one of a series, is the information presented in the same sequence in each table and are the tables named in a parallel fashion?
- Do the tables/figures have a title (a summary of precisely what the figure/table contains)? Do they have an acknowledgement – and do they require one?
- Does every column in a table have a heading?
- Are the tables and figures easily understandable?
- Are tables too large/complex? Could they be turned round or divided into two tables?
- Are the tables too small? Could the information be put in the text (unless the data are very important). Can several small tables be combined?
- Are all values explained?
- Are numbers given to an appropriate degree of accuracy? For example, in a sample of 40, percentages calculated to 2 decimal points are pointless.
- Are percentages correctly calculated? Do the numbers in the tables add up accurately?
- Are the scales in figures the same?
- Do graphs have clear x and y axis definitions?

Discussion

- Are the main findings stated concisely, and is an answer given to the question posed?
- Is the validity of results assessed and any shortcomings in the methods highlighted?
- Are the results compared with other published findings: not to excess and only those relevant?
- Are any results that do not "fit in" discussed?
- Are the significance and implications of the findings discussed?
- Are unanswered questions and future research mentioned?

References

- Are only references that have direct bearing on the work described given?
- Are they up to date? Are they too many/too few?
- Are there any/too many book references, personal communications and unpublished reports?
- Are references correctly and completely cited?

- Are all references mentioned in the text (and not in the abstract) and are they correctly cited and numbered in the text?

Proof checks

General

- Ensure the page layout is correct.
- Check headers/footers are correct (read the header for errors – check it against the title and author names as relevant).
- Read all headings. Check they are all correct and the correct level and the spacing is correct.
- Check contents list against article titles and page numbers.
- Check paragraph ends are properly closed (not justified to the end with rest of paragraph).
- Check spacing between paragraphs, between headings, headings and text and between lines is correct and consistent.
- Check footnotes are correctly/consistently numbered and none is missing.
- Check line spacing on footnotes is proportionate to smaller font size (not as main text).
- If text is more than one column, check column alignment is consistent.
- Look at use of white space: too much or too little?

Figures

- Reread all labels/numbers/words.
- Check it is the correct figure in relation to the text.
- Check they are appropriately placed (as far as possible at the top or bottom of the page as soon after the text reference as possible).
- Check photographs are appropriately placed, well aligned, well sized and do not interfere with readability of text.

Tables and mathematical content

- Check the spacing of rows, and text within rows.
- Check column headings are placed correctly.
- Ensure all column and row alignments are correct.
- Check they are appropriately placed (as far as possible at the top or bottom of the page as soon after the text reference as possible).
- Check specific symbols have correctly converted from one program to another (e.g. ≤ μ χ α β).

Additional Resources

Chicago manual of style, 15th ed. Chicago, University of Chicago Press, 2003.

Council of Science Editors, Style Manual Committee. *Scientific style and format: the CSE manual for authors, editors, and publishers*, 7th ed. Reston, VA, The Council, 2006.

Maisonneuve J et al. (eds). *Science editors' handbook*. UK, European Association of Science Editors (EASE), 2007.

Nadziejka DE. *Levels of technical editing*. Council of Biology Editors, 1999.

O'Conner PT. *Woe is I: the grammarphobe's guide to better English in plain English*, 3rd ed. New York, Riverhead Books, 2004.

Utiger RD. *Syllabus for prospective and newly appointed editors*. USA, The World Association of Medical Editors (WAME), 2001. Visited 29 June 2009. http://www.wame.org/syllabus.htm